The Pediatric Nurse's Survival Guide

The Pediatric Nurse's Survival Guide

Third Edition

Lisa M. Rebeschi, RN, MSN, CNE

Assistant Professor
Department of Nursing
Southern Connecticut State University
New Haven, Connecticut

Mary Heiens Brown, PhD, RN, CPNP

Assistant Professor of Clinical Nursing
University of Texas at Houston
Health Science Center School of Nursing
Houston, Texas

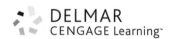
DELMAR
CENGAGE Learning

Australia • Brazil • Japan • Korea • Mexico • Singapore • Spain • United Kingdom • United States

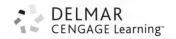
DELMAR
CENGAGE Learning™

The Pediatric Nurse's Survival Guide, Third Edition

Lisa M. Rebeschi, Mary Heiens Brown

Vice President, Health Care Business Unit: William Brottmiller

Director of Learning Solutions: Matthew Kane

Acquisitions Editor: Maureen Rosener

Senior Product Manager: Elisabeth F. Williams

Editorial Assistant: Chelsey Iaquinta

Marketing Director: Jennifer McAvey

Marketing Manager: Michele McTighe

Channel Manager: Danielle Pacella

Technology Director: Laurie K. Davis

Production Director: Carolyn Miller

Content Project Manager: David Buddle

For product information and technology assistance, contact us at **Cengage Learning Customer & Sales Support, 1-800-354-9706**

For permission to use material from this text or product, submit all requests online at **www.cengage.com/permissions** Further permissions questions can be emailed to **permissionrequest@cengage.com**

Library of Congress Control Number:-2006045523

ISBN-13: 978-1-4018-9716-1

ISBN-10: 1-4018-9716-9

Delmar
Executive Woods, 5 Maxwell Drive
Clifton Park, NY 12065, USA

Cengage Learning is a leading provider of customized learning solutions with office locations around the globe, including Singapore, the United Kingdom, Australia, Mexico, Brazil, and Japan. Locate your local office at **international .cengage.com/region**

Cengage Learning products are represented in Canada by Nelson Education, Ltd.

For your course and learning solutions, visit **delmar .cengage.com**

Visit our corporate website at **www.cengage.com**

Notice to the Reader

Printed in the United States of America
4 5 6 7 11 10 09 08

To my husband, Joseph, for providing me with your support and encouragement throughout all of my professional endeavors. To my wonderful toddler, Joey, for all that you have taught me over the past three years.

LMR

CONTENTS

CHAPTER 4
DRUG ADMINISTRATION 83

CHAPTER 5
ESSENTIAL CLINICAL SKILLS 173

CHAPTER 6
COMMON HEALTH PROBLEMS 188

PREFACE

The Pediatric Nurse's Survival Guide, third edition, is a concise pocket-size reference that includes applicable clinical information about laboratory values, common disorders, and medications commonly used with pediatric clients, as well as handy assessment information. *The Pediatric Nurse's Survival Guide* is designed to accompany any core pediatric textbook, or it can be used alone by practicing nurses who need a quick reference.

This third edition includes an expanded section on common health problems of the pediatric client. New additions include information on administration of oxygen, use of restraints, nasotracheal suctioning, tracheostomy care, measuring PEFR, nebulized medications, urinary catheterization, appendicitis, celiac disease, Crohn's disease, and diabetes mellitus. The authors have included common nursing diagnoses found with each health problem. Nursing diagnoses have been updated to reflect *Nursing Diagnoses: Definitions and Classification 2005–2006* by North American Nursing Diagnosis Association. New figures have been added, as well as information on common injection sites, and stages of sexual development. The medication section has been updated to include the medications most commonly given to pediatric clients.

REVIEWERS

Patricia Boyle Egland, RN, MSN, CPNP
Assistant Professor of Pediatric Nursing
City University of New York
Borough of Manhattan Community College
New York, New York

Cara Gallegos, RN, MSN, Doctoral Student
University of New Mexico
Albuquerque, New Mexico

CHAPTER 1

COMMUNICATION

THE NURSING PROCESS AND FAMILY-CENTERED CARE

The nursing process is the framework for professional practice endorsed by the American Nurses Association. The pediatric nurse utilizes the nursing process while caring for hospitalized children and adolescents as a method of problem identification and problem solving. Nonlinear steps of the nursing process consist of assessment, nursing diagnosis, planning, implementation, and evaluation.

- Assessment—provides the foundation for decision making; this continuous process involves collection of subjective and objective data and is holistic in nature
- Nursing Diagnosis—identification of actual or potential problems based on thorough assessment data; results from clustering assessment data; clinical judgment made by the nurse; basis for selection of nursing interventions and outcomes
- Planning—desired outcomes or goals are established in collaboration with the client and family; interventions selected to achieved desired outcomes; plans of care are individualized according to client and family needs
- Implementation—interventions are performed and feedback received
- Evaluation—determine whether goals or outcomes have been achieved; modifications to nursing care plan are made, if necessary

This text utilizes nursing diagnoses approved by the North American Nursing Diagnosis Association (NANDA) for 2005–2006, as well as linkages to current Nursing Outcomes Classification (NOC) and Nursing Interventions Classification (NIC).

While implementing the nursing process with children and families, the nurse also recognizes the need for family-centered care. The philosophy of family-centered care is widely accepted by other health care disciplines and is often integrated in the health care institution's mission and philosophy. Throughout the nursing process the family is supported and acknowledged for its unique strengths. The family is viewed as the "expert" caregiver for the child. With this philosophy of care, the nurse and parent form a partnership while caring for the child. Family-centered care is deliberate in nature; collaboration with the family occurs throughout the nursing process. The following eight elements of family-centered care are essential: the family at the center, family-professional collaboration, family-professional communication, cultural diversity of families, coping differences and support, family-centered peer support, specialized service and support systems, and a holistic perspective of family-centered care. The Institute for Family Centered Care (http://www.familycenteredcare.org) is a particularly useful resource for nurses interested in fully implementing this philosophy of care.

Bill of Rights for Children and Teens

The Association for the Care of Children's Health has published a pediatric bill of rights employed by many pediatric hospitals. Specifically, children and families have the right to:

- Respect and personal dignity
- Supportive care
- Information presented in an understandable manner
- Quality health care
- Emotional support
- Care that respects the need to grow, play, and learn
- Make choices and decisions

COMMUNICATING WITH CHILDREN AND FAMILIES

Communication skills are essential in providing quality nursing care. Nurses need to frequently assess perceptions to assess levels of understanding. Effective communication in the pediatric setting requires communication skills with both children and their caregiver(s).

Some of the basic principles to keep in mind are the following:

- Remember that privacy is an essential component
- Properly identify yourself, your role, and your purpose
- Ensure confidentiality, including maintaining safeguards for privacy of computerized client data
- Be aware of environmental characteristics
- Begin communication with more general content before getting specific
- Communicate directly with the child even when accompanied by an adult
- Remember that adolescents may need to communicate in private without the presence of family members

- Use open-ended questions appropriately
- Encourage continued communication with nonverbal gestures such as nodding and eye contact
- Recognize and be respectful of cultural influences on communication
- Use trained interpreters as necessary, rather than bilingual family members or friends
- Remember that silence is an appropriate communication technique
- Remember that active listening to both nonverbal and verbal cues is one of the most important components of effective communication
- Ensure mutual understanding by restating the therapeutic communication technique
- Avoid common communication blockers such as changing focus, falsely reassuring, interrupting, forming prejudged conclusions, and overloading with information
- Maintain eye-level position with child during communication
- Remember that transition objects such as stuffed animals may be useful when communicating with children
- Remember that writing, drawing, and playing are alternative communication approaches for older children
- Remember that honesty is of ultimate importance

Sign Language

Children with cognitive or sensory impairments often use American Sign Language (ASL) to communicate with others. Sign language utilizes visual gestures, movements, and hand signals for communication instead of verbal words. Most nurses and other health care providers do not have ASL skills. During periods of hospitalization, this may provide for difficult communication with the child. Although there are many published ASL references, they are not usually readily available in the acute care setting. The website "American Sign Language Browser" http://commtechlab. msu.edu is a useful online reference for nurses who need to communicate with the child who signs. The site provides video clips of thousands of ASL signs.

CULTURALLY SENSITIVE APPROACHES

Nurses are continually challenged to meet the needs of a multicultural society as they provide care to diverse populations. Nurses recognize that culture plays an important role in the socialization of children and that cultural values are passed from one generation to the next by the family unit. A holistic view of children and families requires an understanding and respect of cultural influences.

Culture provides children and families with a sort of "blueprint" for living, thinking, behaving, and feeling. It guides the way in which individuals solve their problems and derive meaning from their lives.

To provide culturally sensitive care, nurses must evaluate their own feelings, prejudices, and beliefs. Nurses must make a conscious effort to recognize, appreciate, and respect differing views and beliefs of clients. Cultural sensitivity involves an awareness of both cultural similarities and differences.

The following are some general guidelines to follow in relation to cultural sensitivity:

- Avoid generalizations about ethnic groups because they may not apply
- Allow children and caregivers to select their own comfortable distance (also use this guide when touching clients)
- Observe family interactions to determine acceptable and appropriate gestures
- Observe cues regarding appropriate eye contact
- Always ask for clarification when uncertain
- Use positive tone of voice to convey genuine interest
- Encourage questions
- Learn basic words, gestures, and beliefs when a family's culture or language is different from your own
- Use information written in the family's native language
- Continually evaluate your own values and beliefs regarding other cultures
- Address intergenerational needs as family members may need to consult with others

It is essential to understand communication patterns of various cultural groups in order to preserve the values, norms, beliefs, and practices of each particular culture. It is true that the process of communication is universal. However, the use of silence, facial expressions, eye and head movements, body posture, and touch may be culturally unique. Although there is much variation even within cultures, the following provides some *general* information regarding communication styles of various cultural groups. The following information should be used as a starting reference and the reader should not generalize these communication characteristics to all members of a cultural group. It is essential to realize that there is as much, if not more, variation within cultures than there is across cultural groups.

Cultural Group	Communication Styles
Asian American	Nonverbal cues very important; silence valued; touching limited; may be hesitant to ask questions; may smile when something is not understood; direct eye contact may be viewed as disrespectful; stoic with emotions

Cultural Group	Communication Styles
African Americans	Value direct eye contact; expressive use of nonverbal behaviors
Haitians	Hand gesturing commonly used; smiling and nodding in agreement may not indicate understanding; direct eye contact used; touch appreciated and seen as comforting
Hispanic Americans	Physical introductory embrace is common; *prolonged* eye contact viewed as disrespectful; relaxed sense of time; in times of stress, tend to revert to native language
Native Americans	Nonverbal communication important; silence is essential component of communication; hesitant to discuss personal situation unless trusting relationship is established
Middle Eastern	Do not shake hands outside immediate family relationship; use silence as show of respect
White Americans	Nod to communicate understanding; handshake; smiling and quiet speaking indicate good social manners

THE USE OF PLAY IN CHILDREN

Play is described as the "work" of children. It is crucial to maintain the activities of play with children who are hospitalized. Play serves several functions: sensorimotor development, intellectual development, socialization, moral development, creative outlets, avenue for self-awareness, and therapeutic value.

TOY SAFETY TIPS

During hospitalization, it is essential to ensure the safety of the child by determining the safety of the child's playthings. This is also important information to include as part of your teaching with families and other caregivers.

- Because foreign body aspiration is the most common cause of toy-related deaths, it is important to assess for any choking hazards. Toys with small parts should absolutely be avoided with any child under the age of 3 (this includes small balls as these can occlude the child's airway). Parents should be taught that any toy that can fit in a toilet paper roll is too small for a child under the age of 3.
- When using balls with children under the age of 6, be certain that the diameter of the ball is greater than 1.75 inches.
- Although children love balloons, latex balloons are not safe for children under the age of 8 (mylar type balloons are a safer alternative).

- Mobiles should not be used in the crib of a child over the age of 5 months or with children who can push up on their hands and knees.
- Pull toys should be examined; the length of cord should be less than 8 inches.
- Toys are generally labeled with the intended age group. Just because the toy is safe for one age group does not mean it is safe for all.
- Be certain that art supplies do not contain toxic chemicals; products should clearly be labeled as nontoxic.
- Avoid toys that produce loud noises as these may be damaging to the child's hearing.
- Protective gear (e.g., helmets, padding) should be worn at all times when using riding-type toys.
- Toys should routinely be inspected for loose parts and other potential hazards.
- Stay abreast of toy recalls from the Consumer Product Safety Commission by accessing the website http://www.recalls.gov.

The following suggestions are play activities by age for children who are hospitalized.

Infants
- Colorful mobiles
- Music boxes
- Mirrors
- Infant swing
- Colored blocks
- Nested boxes or cups
- Large picture books

Toddlers
- Sing-along CDs or audiotapes
- Pull toys
- Riding toys (e.g., ride-on cars, trucks, rocking horse)
- Wooden puzzles
- Finger paints
- Coloring with thick crayons
- Play dough
- Stuffed animals, dolls (check for safety)
- Television, videos, interactive computer games

Preschoolers

- Riding toys (e.g., tricycle)
- Puppets
- Drawing, coloring, cutting out pictures
- Scrapbooking
- Dolls, stuffed animals
- Dress up
- Jigsaw puzzles
- Books
- Musical toys
- Finger paints

School-Age Children

- Card playing
- Board games
- Drawing
- Movies, videos
- Interactive video games
- Play involving peer interaction

Adolescents

- Board games
- Audiotapes, CDs, radio
- Videos, movies
- Mental challenge games
- Craft activities

Therapeutic play may be used when the child is unable to completely verbalize his or her feelings. It is used to better understand the child's thoughts about hospitalization, procedures, fears, and concerns. Both verbal and nonverbal messages from the child are important. Drawing, painting, anatomically correct dolls, and direct play with medical equipment are often used. The following are some general guidelines for therapeutic play:

- Allow as much choice as possible for children to select articles to play with
- Allow the child to play with actual medical materials that he or she will be confronted with (e.g., stethoscope, nasogastric [NG] tube, tympanic thermometer)
- Use therapeutic communication techniques
- Ask the child to describe his or her drawings
- Always supervise therapeutic play
- Consult with child life therapists if available

CHAPTER 2

ASSESSMENT

PHYSICAL ASSESSMENT
General Guidelines

The physical assessment of a pediatric client should be performed as opportunities present. Therefore, be prepared with all equipment, including stethoscope, tape measure, penlight, and tongue blade, when entering a client's room. The assessment should begin immediately. The client's skin color, position, and gait (if the child is observed walking) should be noted, as well as the caregiver's response and caregiver-child interaction. If an infant is sleeping, it is a good time to listen to his or her heart sounds. Rapport and trust can be established with the caregiver and child by talking with both the caregiver and the child. If the nurse has to leave the room to retrieve forgotten equipment, rapport with the child will have to be reestablished.

The nurse can use play therapy as necessary to accomplish his or her assessment of the child. For example, listening to the caregiver's or a stuffed toy's heart and lungs can show children, especially toddlers, that it does not hurt. The nurse can then attempt to obtain resting heart rate, heart sounds, respirations, and breath sounds. The child also can be allowed to assist with the assessment as he or she is able. Preschoolers and older children like to listen to their own heart sounds. This is a valuable opportunity to teach a child about the body and how to keep it healthy, as well as to validate the child's normalcy. Other general guidelines to consider include involving the child as much as possible in the assessment process. For example, provide choices for the child to make; they may choose whether to be examined while lying in bed or sitting in a parent's lap. Children also appreciate being able to handle the necessary assessment equipment, such as the stethoscope, otoscope, tongue blades, and so on. It is also important to explain what you are doing to the child in age-appropriate language. Reassurance and praise throughout the assessment may enhance the child's cooperation.

Invasive procedures and painful areas or procedures should be saved until the end of the assessment. What constitutes invasive varies with age groups. For example, examining the ears, mouth, and nose is invasive to toddlers.

Genitourinary system and abdominal procedures are invasive to school-age children and adolescents. If the child refuses to cooperate, the nurse must use a firm approach and perform the examination as quickly as possible. Regardless of the order in which the assessment is performed, it must be charted in a logical head-to-toe format. Health care institutions usually have institution-specific documentation forms for recording assessment findings.

General Appearance

Note the overall impression of the child. For example, does the child appear happy, sad, or frightened; small, obese, or well nourished; awake, alert, cooperative, developmentally appropriate for age, lethargic, or distressed? What is the client's state of consciousness? Observations of general appearance take place throughout the assessment. It is important to note the child's facial appearance as this may provide clues regarding the child's condition (i.e., level of pain or discomfort, dyspnea). Observations of hygiene and condition of clothing can provide clues to potential instances of child abuse, neglect, or lack of financial resources.

Skin

Inspect and palpate the skin for color. (Remember that room color, gown color, and lighting affect observation. Evaluate for jaundice in natural lighting of a window; cyanosis blanches momentarily, bruises do not.) Also note pigmentation, temperature, texture, moisture, and turgor.

Note and describe all lesions for the following:

Location—exactly where on body
Pattern—clustered, confluent, evanescent, linear
Size—measured in centimeters
Color—red, pink, brown, white, hyperpigmented, or hypopigmented
Elevation—raised (papular), flat (macular), fluid filled (vesicular)
Blanching—do they pale when pressure is applied?

Because the incidence of skin cancer in children is on the rise, it is essential to accurately assess skin lesions. The ABCDE mnemonic is helpful when assessing the child with skin lesions. Specifically observe for:

- **A**symmetry (i.e., one half is different than the other)
- **B**order irregularity
- **C**olor (lesion varies in color)
- **D**iameter greater than 6 millimeters
- **E**levation

Level of hydration is also assessed with the skin. Tissue turgor (elasticity) can be assessed by pulling the skin on the child's abdomen between your thumb and index finger and then quickly releasing it. Tissue should resume normal position immediately and not leave any creases. Children who are dehydrated may demonstrate "tenting" of skin or slow return of skin to its normal position. Along with the monitoring of the child's weight, skin turgor is one of the best estimates of normal hydration.

Edema should also be noted if present. To check for edema, imprint your thumb firmly against the tibia or ankle malleolus. Normally, the skin tissue should remain smooth. If your pressure leaves a skin indentation, note this as *pitting edema*. Grade the amount of pitting on a 4-point scale as follows:

- 1+—mild or slight indentation with no notable swelling of the leg
- 2+—moderate indentation subsides rapidly
- 3+—deep pitting with indentation remaining for a short time; leg looks swollen
- 4+—very deep pitting with lasting indentation and a very swollen leg

Hair

Note the hair's color, texture, distribution, quality, and loss. Look in hair behind the ears for nits. Hair should appear well-distributed, shiny, and firmly attached to the scalp.

Nails

Note the color, cyanosis, shape, and condition of nails. Clubbing is determined by checking nail angle. The normal angle is 160 degrees. An angle of 180 degrees or larger is seen in clubbing caused by long-term hypoxia.

Head

Inspect the head for shape and symmetry and palpate the child's head, feeling for bogginess, sutures, and fontanels. The posterior fontanel normally closes from birth to 2 months and is usually 1 to 2 cm in size. The anterior fontanel normally closes between 9 and 18 months but should be closed by 2 years. Measure the anterior fontanel in two dimensions; usually it is 4 to 5 cm by 3 to 4 cm, but should be at least 1 cm by 1 cm. Normally, the fontanels should feel flat. In states of dehydration, fontanels may be sunken. In states of increased intracranial pressure, fontanels may be bulging. Measure frontal occipital circumference (FOC) until the child is 36 months old or if its size is important to the child's condition after 2 years of age. Always plot FOC and note the size, shape, and symmetry of the head. Palpate the scalp for tenderness and lesions.

Neck

Inspect the neck for swelling, webbing, nuchal fold, and vein distension. Palpate for swelling, carotid pulse, trachea, and thyroid.

Ears

Inspect the ears for shape, color, symmetry, helix formation, and position or placement. The top of the ear should go through an imaginary line from the inner canthus to the outer canthus to the occiput. Palpate for firmness and pain and observe for and describe any discharge from the ear canal. Expected findings from otoscopic examination include pearly gray color of the tympanic membrane, cone-shaped light reflex at the 5 or 7 o'clock position, and appearance of bony landmarks. Assess for gross hearing. Infants less than 4 months of age startle to sound. Older infants turn to localize the sound of jingling keys and other objects. Use the whisper test, Rinne test, and Weber test with verbal and cooperative children.

Eyes

Inspect the eyes for position, alignment, lid closure, inner canthal distance (average = 2.5 cm), epicanthal folds, and slant of fissure. Note dark circles under the eyes (usually present in children with allergies).

Brows—note separateness, nits
Lashes—note if they curve into eye
Lids—note color, swelling, lesions, discharge
Conjunctiva
    Palpebral (should be pink)—note redness, pallor
    Sclera and bulbar—note injection, redness, color (should be white; yellow in jaundice, blue in osteogenesis imperfecta)
Pupils—note shape, size, and briskness of reaction to light by constricting directly and consensually and accommodation for near and far vision
Iris—note color, roundness, any clefts or defects
Extraocular movements (EOMs)
    Six cardinal fields of gaze—Hold child's chin and have him or her follow your finger, moving in the shape of an H, with his or her eyes to note asymmetric eye movement or to elicit nystagmus; a few beats of nystagmus in the far lateral gaze are normal.
    Corneal light reflex—Hold light 15 inches from the bridge of the nose and shine on the bridge. It should reflect in the same place in each eye in normally aligned eyes.
    Cover-uncover test—Check for movement when one eye is covered and the other is gazing at a distant object. Remove the cover and note movement of the covered eye. Repeat using a near object.
    Gross vision—Newborns blink and hyperextend their necks to light. Infants who can see fix on and follow objects. Grossly assess older children's vision by having them describe what they see on the wall or out the window.

Face

Note the color, symmetrical movement, expression, skin folds, and swelling of the face.

Nose

Inspect the nose for color of skin, any nasal crease, nasal mucosa, any discharge and its color, and patency. Flaring of nares may be a sign of respiratory distress. Assess turbinates by shining a light into the nares while pushing up gently on the tip of the nose (red and swollen indicates possible upper respiratory infection; pale and boggy indicates possible allergic rhinitis). Infants are obligate nose breathers until approximately 3 months of age. Palpate sinuses for tenderness. Frontal sinuses are not developed completely until approximately 8 years of age.

Mouth

Inspect all areas of the mouth. Note the number and condition of teeth. To calculate the expected number of teeth in infants, subtract 6 from the infant's age in months (e.g., 12 months − 6 = 6 teeth). Observe tonsils for swelling (grade 1+ indicates mild swelling; grade 4+ indicates touching, or "kissing," tonsils), color (should be same color as buccal mucosa), and discharge. Examine and palpate the hard and soft palate for color, patency, and lesions. The uvula should rise symmetrically; a bifid uvula could indicate a submucosal cleft. Note tongue shape, size, color, and movement, and inspect for any lesions (most common lesions are white and are thrush). Note breath odor.

Thorax and Lungs

Inspect for symmetry, movement, color, retractions, breast development, and type and effort of breathing. Breathing is predominately abdominal until age 7. Note nasal flaring and use of accessory muscles. Retractions usually start subcostal and substernal, then progress to suprasternal and supraclavicular, and lastly intercostal, indicating severe distress. Palpate for tactile fremitus (increased in congestion and consolidation). Percuss for resonance (sound becomes dull with fluid or masses). Auscultate side to side for symmetry of sound. Infants breathe deeper when they cry; toddlers and preschoolers can breathe deeper when they blow bubbles or try to "blow out the light" of your pen light. Assess all fields. Listen to the back to assess the lower lobes in children younger than 8. Auscultate in the axillae to best hear crackles in children with suspected pneumonia. Normal sounds are vesicular or bronchovesicular. Infants' breath sounds are louder and more bronchial because they have thin chest walls.

Describe adventitious sounds as follows:

Rhonchi—a continuous, low-pitched sound with a snoring quality
Crackles—intermittent, brief, repetitive sounds caused by small collapsed
    airways popping open
    Fine crackles—soft, high-pitched, and brief
    Coarse crackles—louder, lower-pitched, and slightly longer than fine
        crackles
Wheezes—musical, more continuous sounds produced by rapid move-
    ment of air through narrowed passages
    Usual progression of wheezing starts with expiratory wheezes only,
        then inspiratory wheezes with decreased expiratory wheezes, then
        inspiratory wheezes only (airways are collapsing on expiration), and
        finally, no sounds because there is little air movement.
Stridor—inspiratory wheeze heard louder in neck than in chest, usually
    right over trachea

Infants with upper airway congestion can have sounds transmitted to lungs
because they are obligate nose breathers. Listen to their lungs when they are
crying and breathing through their mouths to decrease the amount of transmitted noise and better assess their breath sounds.

Cardiovascular System

Inspect for point of maximum impulse (PMI), cyanosis, mottling (uneveness
in color), edema, respiratory distress, clubbing, activity intolerance, and tiring with feeds. Palpate PMI and brachial, radial, femoral, and pedal pulses.

Auscultate the following areas with the bell and diaphragm of the stethoscope:

Aortic area	Right second intercostal space (ICS) at right sternal border (SB)
Pulmonic area	Left second ICS at left SB
Erb's point	Left third ICS at left SB
Tricuspid	Left fifth ICS at left SB
Mitral	Left fifth ICS at left midclavicular line

S_1 correlates with the carotid pulse and is best heard at the apex of the heart.
S_2 is best heard in the aortic and pulmonic areas (base of heart). Quality of
sound should be crisp and clear. Heart rate should be normal for age and
condition and synchronous with the radial pulse. Rhythm should be regular
or may slow and speed up with respirations in young infants. Auscultate with
the child in two positions if possible. Auscultate for muffled or additional
sounds and note where these are best heard.

Murmurs should be assessed for the following:

Location—where heard best on the chest wall

Timing in cardiac cycle—continuous, systolic, or diastolic

Grade—I/VI to VI/VI

    I/VI—very faint, have to really tune in

    II/VI—quiet, but can hear soon after placing stethoscope

    III/VI—moderately loud

    IV/VI—loud

    V/VI—very loud, may be heard with stethoscope partially off chest

    VI/VI—can hear without stethoscope

Pitch—high (best heard with the diaphragm), medium, or low (best heard with the bell)

Quality—harsh, blowing, machinery-like, musical

Radiation—does it radiate, and if so where (listen to back, axillae, and above clavicles)

Abdomen

Inspect the abdomen for pulsation, contour, symmetry, peristaltic waves, masses, and normal skin color. Auscultate before palpating so that normal bowel sounds are not disturbed. Listen in all four quadrants for a full minute. Normal sounds should be heard every 10 to 30 seconds; you should hear 4 to 5 sounds per minute. Less than 4 per minute indicates decreased bowel sounds. Listen for a full 5 minutes before concluding that they are absent.

Percuss for dullness over the client's liver and full bladder. The rest of the abdomen should percuss tympani. Palpate using light pressure first. Have the child bend the knees up while lying on his or her back to relax the abdomen. Use the child's hands under your hands if the child is very ticklish or tense. With deep palpation, support the child from the back, then palpate. Start in lower quadrants and move upward to detect an enlarged liver or spleen. Note areas of tenderness, pain, or any masses.

Anus

Inspect the skin and perineum for excoriation, bruising, discoloration, or tears.

Genitourinary System

    Female genitalia—Note redness, excoriation, discharge, and odor.

    Male genitalia—Note if circumcised or uncircumcised. (If uncircumcised, see if foreskin is retractable.) Note position of meatus. Close off the canals and feel for the testes or any masses in the scrotal sac. If you feel a mass other than the testes, transilluminate for fluid. Hydroceles are fluid in the scrotal sac and will transilluminate light. Hernias are loops of bowel and will not transilluminate.

Lymphatic System

Palpate the lymphatic system throughout the examination with the pads of the fingers. Nodes should be firm, small (1 cm or less), freely moveable, and nontender. Palpate preauricular, postauricular, anterior and posterior cervical chains, supraclavicular and subclavicular, axillary, and inguinal lymph nodes.

Musculoskeletal System

Incorporate assessment of the musculoskeletal system into the rest of the examination. Observe walking, sitting, turning, and range of motion in all joints. Observe spinal curvature and mobility. Exaggerated lumbar curve is normal in toddlers. Note sacral dimples or tufts of hair at the base of the spinal column. Note symmetry and movement of the extremities.

Test muscle strength. Strength is graded on a 0 to 5 scale. Normal muscle strength is grade 5.

0—no contraction noted
1—barely a trace of contraction
2—active movement without gravity
3—active movement against gravity
4—active movement against gravity and resistance
5—active movement against full resistance without tiring

Note size, color, temperature, and mobility of joints. Examine palmar creases. A single crease is a *simian crease* and can be associated with Down syndrome. Note extra digits and deformities. Thumb deformities may be associated with heart defects.

Note stance and gait. Bowed legs (genu varum) are normal in toddlers until approximately age 2. Knock-knees (genu valgum) are normal from age 2 until approximately 6 to 10. Note foot deformities. Stroke the side of the foot to see if it returns to a neutral position. Check for dislocatable hips using Barlow's test and the Ortolani maneuver. Also look for uneven skin folds.

Nervous System

Observe grossly for speech and ability to follow directions in an older child. In an infant, observe activity and tone. In ambulatory patients, observe gait and balance.

Use a percussion hammer or the side of the stethoscope diaphragm to elicit the following responses:

Deep Tendon Reflex	Procedure	Response
Biceps	Hit antecubital space	Forearm flexes
Triceps	Bend arm at elbow, hit triceps tendon above elbow	Forearm extends
Patellar	Strike patellar tendon	Lower leg extends
Achilles	Hold foot lightly, hit Achilles tendon	Foot flexes downward
Cranial nerves	Most are integrated into routine examination and are not specifically tested.	

Check deep tendon reflexes. These are graded from 0 to 4+.

4+—very brisk, hyperactive
3+—brisker than average
2+—normal
1+—decreased
0—absent

Infant Reflexes	Age	Assessment
Babinski	Birth to 2 yr	Stroke bottom of foot; toes fan
Galant	Birth to 4–8 wk	Stroke infant's side; hips swing to that side
Moro	Birth to 3–4 mo	Arms extend, fingers fan (if asymmetrical, brachial plexus injury should be suspected); if Moro persists beyond 6 mo, brain damage should be suspected
Palmar grasp	Birth to 4 mo	Put your finger in infant's palm from ulnar side; infant closes fingers around your finger
Rooting	Birth to 4 mo (up to 12 mo during sleep)	Stroke infant's cheek and corner of mouth; infant's head turns in that direction
Sucking	Birth to 4 mo (7 mo during sleep)	Infant has reflexive sucking to stimuli

Neurovascular System

Assess the neurovascular system very closely in children with intravenous (IV) lines in extremities, and those in casts, restraints, and in traction. Note color and size of extremity and compare with unaffected extremity.

Check pulses bilaterally for equality of strength. Check capillary refill time by pinching a toe or finger and noting the time it takes for the color to return. They should have brisk, immediate blood return. Both congestive heart failure and dehydration can increase capillary refill time. Assess for any alterations in sensation or increased pain.

NEONATAL VARIANCES IN ASSESSMENT

General

Note overall impression (e.g., alert, awake, sleepy, responsive). Note cry intensity and pitch. A high-pitched cry is associated with increased intracranial pressure.

Skin

Color (assess before disturbing)

Plethora —ruddy, red color associated with a high hematocrit

Acrocyanosis—cyanosis of the hands and feet; normal in first few days

Jaundice—yellow color; common after first 24 hr; assess in natural light (In dark skin clients, assess mucous membranes and sclera for jaundice)

Bruising—common with difficult deliveries; facial bruising common in face presentations and in infants with nuchal cords (cord around the neck)

Petechiae—normal on face and upper trunk in rapid deliveries

Cyanosis—assess for cause (cyanosis will blanch, bruises will not)

Pustular melanosis—small pustules at birth that reveal freckles when burst; common finding in infants with dark skin; persists approximately 3 to 4 months

Erythema toxicum neonaterum—"normal newborn rash"; evanescent rash characterized by small yellow pustules on an erythematous base; most common in infants with fair skin; usually appears after first 24 hr and lasts up to 2 weeks

Peeling skin—associated with postmaturity

Milia—small white dots usually present on nose or chin; caused by blocked sweat glands; resolve by 2 to 4 months

Nevus flammeus—"stork bites," also called salmon patches; most commonly on the nape of the neck and eyelids; turn bright red when infant cries; usually fade over the first year

Mongolian spots—normal hyperpigmented areas most commonly seen in infants with dark skin; usually on sacral area, but can be anywhere; may be purple, blue, green, or brown

Hair

Note whorls and abnormal coloring or distribution of hair. Color may change. Infants lose initial hair, which is replaced with permanent hair during the first 6 months. Some lose it gradually, and some all at once. In fact, bald spots from rubbing the head on the mattress are common.

Nails

Infants' nails may be meconium stained. The longer the nails, the more mature the infant.

Head

Note anterior and posterior fontanels. They may appear larger than normal because of open sagittal or frontal sutures. This is not of concern if FOC is normal. Sutures may override as a result of molding to fit in the birth canal. Sutures should be flat by 6 months. Measure and plot FOC to determine microcephaly or hydrocephaly. Note electrode marks and observe them daily for infection.

Caput succedaneum—diffuse swelling, usually over occiput, that crosses suture lines and is usually resolved in the first few days

Cephalohematoma—distinct swelling that does not cross suture lines; caused by bleeding into the periosteum; calcifies then absorbs; persists about 3–4 months

Craniotabes—a "ping-pong ball" effect of the bone usually caused by thin cranial bones; normal near the sutures, abnormal where the bones should be thick; can be indicative of hydrocephaly or syphilis

Neck

The neck is usually short. Note webbing (common in Turner's syndrome) and nuchal folds (normal variation in large infants or associated with other findings in Down syndrome).

Ears

Note the position of the ears. Low-set ears are associated with renal abnormalities and hearing loss. A rolled or flat helix usually is a result of intrauterine position. Assess for gross hearing. Newborns should blink to loud noises (acoustical blink reflex). Note preauricular pits and tags. Pits usually are not significant, but large tags can be associated with hearing problems.

Eyes

Note the position and alignment of the eyes. Note red reflex bilaterally. Cloudy red reflex is associated with congenital cataracts. White reflexes are associated with retinoblastoma. Red reflexes in infants with dark skin are not bright red, but rather a more pinkish-gray as a result of pigment. Lids may be puffy because of chemical conjunctivitis caused by prophylactic drops given at birth. Short palpebral fissures may be associated with fetal alcohol syndrome.

Face

The infant's face may be asymmetrical because of intrauterine position. Assess for symmetry of movement, especially if forceps were used during delivery. Note abnormal facial features.

Nose

The infant's nose may be asymmetrical because of intrauterine position. Assess for patency. Infants are obligate nose breathers until 3 months of age.

Mouth

Assess the palate and suck and gag reflexes. Note any natal teeth. A large tongue may be associated with hypothyroidism and Down syndrome. Note any ankyloglossia (tongue-tie); this may interfere with successful breastfeeding and speech acquisition if the tongue is too tightly anchored to the floor of the mouth.

Thorax and Lungs

Breast engorgement with or without milky discharge is normal in both sexes and is associated with maternal hormones. This resolves without intervention but may persist for up to 6 months, or longer in breastfed infants. Supranummary or extra nipples are common. These will not develop further.

A newborn's xiphoid process curves upward and normally is very prominent. Breath sounds should be equal bilaterally and usually sound louder because of a thin chest wall. Note tachypnea (respiratory rate >60), grunting, flaring, and retractions.

Cardiovascular System

Assess an infant's cardiovascular system as with an older child. Grades II to III/VI murmers are common at the upper left sternal border (LSB); continuous sound usually indicates a patent ductus arteriosus. Systolic murmurs at the upper LSB usually are transient and benign. Murmurs at the mid-LSB or lower LSB bear watching. Compare brachial and femoral pulses. If femoral pulses are diminished or absent, check and compare blood pressures from the four extremities.

Abdomen

The umbilical cord should have three vessels (two arteries and one vein). The cord should be treated with alcohol and should dry and fall off within the first 3 weeks. Umbilical hernias are present in 90% of newborns and are normal. Note the size of any defects in the abdominal wall. If the rectus muscle is not fused at birth, the infant has diastasis recti. This is a normal finding and usually closes by itself during the first year. The liver normally is palpated at the costal margin or down 2 cm; in preterm infants it should not be palpated down more than half way to the umbilicus. The spleen normally is not palpated.

Anus

Check the patency of the anus.

Genitourinary System

   Male—foreskin normally tight and meatus not visualized; testes may be retractile or in the canals

   Female—hypertrophied hymen or hymenal tag caused by maternal hormones is common and recedes as maternal hormonal influence fades; may have clear vaginal discharge that turns white, then bloody like a menstrual period before it goes away; once resolved, it should not return; prominent labial minora is normal in preterm infants

Lymphatic System

Nodes usually are not palpable.

Musculoskeletal System

Feel for crepitus over the clavicles. Fractures are common in large infants. With an asymmetrical Moro reflex, suspect brachial plexus injury. Feel all long bones for crepitus. Note tone. "Floppy" babies with significantly decreased tone need to be assessed further for hypoglycemia, perinatal drug exposure, sepsis, or chromosomal abnormalities.

Nervous System

Check normal infant reflexes. Infants who are jittery need to be assessed for hypoglycemia and perinatal drug exposure.

Normal Vital Signs

NORMAL TEMPERATURES IN CHILDREN

	Temperature (in degrees)	
Age	Fahrenheit	Centigrade
Newborn–1 yr	99.4–99.7	37.5–37.7
3–5 yr	98.6–99.0	37.0–37.2
7–9 yr	98.1–98.3	36.7–36.8
10 yr to adult	97.8	36.6.
	$F = (C \times 9/5) + 32$	$C = (F - 32) \times 5/9$

NORMAL HEART RATES IN CHILDREN

Age	Awake at Rest (bpm)	Asleep (bpm)	Exercise/Fever (bpm)
Newborn	100–180	80–160	up to 220
1 wk to 3 mo	100–220	80–200	up to 220
3 mo to 2 yr	80–150	70–120	up to 200
2 to 10 yr	70–110	60–90	up to 200
10 yr to adult	55–90	50–90	up to 200

bpm, beats per minute.
Adapted from Potts, N. L., & Mandleco, B. L. (2007). *Pediatric nursing: Caring for children and their families* (2nd ed.). Clifton Park, NY: Thomson Delmar Learning.

GRADING OF PULSES

Grade	Description
0	Not palpable
+1	Difficult to palpate; thready; weak; can be easily obliterated with pressure
+2	Difficult to palpate; may be obliterated with pressure
+3	Easy to palpate; not easily obliterated
+4	Strong; bounding; not obliterated with pressure

NORMAL RESPIRATORY RATES FOR CHILDREN

Age	Rate (breaths per minute)	Age	Rate (breaths per minute)
Newborn	35	8 yr	20
1–11 mo	30	10–12 yr	19
2 yr	25	14 yr	18
4 yr	23	16 yr	17
6 yr	21	18 yr	16–18

Adapted from Potts, N. L., & Mandleco, B. L. (2007). *Pediatric nursing: Caring for children and their families* (2nd ed.). Clifton Park, NY: Thomson Delmar Learning.

ASSESSMENT OF NORMAL BREATH SOUNDS

Classification	Description
Vesicular	Heard over entire lung surface, except upper intrascapular area and below manubrium
Bronchovesicular	Heard over manubrium and in upper intrascapular areas where trachea and bronchi bifurcate; inspirations are louder and higher in pitch than in vesicular breathing
Bronchial	Heard only near suprasternal notch over trachea; inspiratory phase is short and expiratory phase is long

NORMAL BLOOD PRESSURE RATES IN CHILDREN (BASED ON 50TH PERCENTILE)

Age	Females		Males	
	Systolic	Diastolic	Systolic	Diastolic
1 day	65	55	73	55
3 days	72	55	74	55
7 days	78	54	76	54
1 mo	84	52	86	52
2 mo	87	51	91	50
3 mo	90	51	91	50
4 mo	90	52	91	50
5 mo	91	52	91	52
6 mo	91	53	90	53
7 mo	91	53	90	54
8 mo	91	53	90	55
9 mo	91	54	90	55
10 mo	91	54	90	56
11 mo	91	54	90	56
1 yr	91	54	90	56
2 yr	90	56	91	56
3 yr	91	56	92	55
4 yr	92	56	93	56
5 yr	94	56	95	56
6 yr	96	57	96	57
7 yr	97	58	97	58
8 yr	99	59	99	60
9 yr	100	61	101	61
10 yr	102	62	102	62
11 yr	105	64	105	63
12 yr	107	66	107	64
13 yr	109	64	109	63

NORMAL BLOOD PRESSURE RATES IN CHILDREN
(BASED ON 50TH PERCENTILE) *(Continued)*

	Females		Males	
Age	Systolic	Diastolic	Systolic	Diastolic
14 yr	110	67	112	64
15 yr	111	67	114	65
16 yr	112	67	117	67
17 yr	112	66	119	69
18 yr	112	66	121	70

Adapted from Potts, N. L., & Mandleco, B. L. (2007). *Pediatric nursing: Caring for children and their families* (2nd ed.). Clifton Park, NY: Thomson Delmar Learning.

Growth Measurements

One of the most important areas in assessing children is the measurement of physical growth. The pediatric nurse should measure weight, height and length, head circumference, skinfold thickness, and arm circumference. Measurements are plotted on growth charts to determine percentiles to compare an individual child's measurements with that of the general population.

The National Center for Health Statistics (NCHS) has developed growth charts according to age. There is one growth chart to be used for children from birth to 36 months of age. In this age group, the weight by age, recumbent length by age, weight for length, and head circumference by age are plotted. There is another growth chart to be used for children ages 2 to 20 years. In this age group, weight by age and stature by age are plotted (see charts on pages 30–31).

The NCHS uses the 5th and 95th percentiles as the parameters for determining if children fall outside of the normal limits for growth. Those below the 5th percentile are considered underweight or small in stature and those above the 95th percentile are considered overweight or large in stature. Children whose measurements fall below or above the 95th percentile should be followed more closely, especially when genetic factors are not involved.

Recumbent length should be measured when the birth to 36-month growth chart is being used. The nurse should fully extend the infant's or child's body. The child should be placed on a papered surface and the nurse should mark the measurements at the top of the head and the heel of the foot. The child is then removed from the surface and the surface is measured with a tape measure.

Height is measured when using the 2 to 20 year growth chart. Height refers to the measurement taken when a child is standing upright. The child's shoes should be removed when measuring height. The head should be in midline and the child should be facing straight forward. There should be no flexion of the knees, slumping of the shoulders, or raising of the heels during the measurement. The most accurate measurements are taken with a wall-mounted stadiometer.

The nurse should use a balanced scale to measure a child's weight. Children should be weighed nude when using the birth to 36-month growth chart. If a child is wearing something heavy, such as a cast or an IV board, that should be documented with the child's weight. When placing the child on an infant scale, the nurse must remember safety issues.

Head circumference is another key growth measurement in children. In general, head circumference is measured from birth to 36 months of age. The measurement should be taken at the greatest circumference, which is slightly above the eyebrows and ear pinna and around the occipital prominence at the back of the skull. A paper tape measure should be used to give the most accurate data.

Chest circumference is measured primarily for comparison with head circumference. Chest circumference is measured at the nipple line midway between inspiration and expiration.

Measuring skinfold thickness is one way to assess body fat. Calipers are used to measure the skinfold thickness in one or more of the following sites: triceps, subscapula, abdomen, upper thigh, and suprailiac. An average of at least two measurements from each site is used.

The measurement of arm circumference is an indirect assessment used to evaluate nutrition. The arm circumference is measured with a paper tape measure, which is placed vertically along the posterior upper arm until the same measurement appears at the acromial process and olecranon process.

NORMAL GROWTH PARAMETERS RELATED TO WEIGHT, HEIGHT, AND HEAD CIRCUMFERENCE

Age	Weight	Height	Head Circumference
1–6 mo	Gains 5–8 oz per wk	Grows 1 inch per mo	Average head circumference is 37–38 cm
7–12 mo	Gains 4–5 oz per wk	Grows ½ inch per mo	
12–18 mo	Gains 2–6 lb in next 6 mo	Grows to 33 inches by 18 mo	Head circumference equals chest circumference at 12 mo

NORMAL GROWTH PARAMETERS RELATED TO WEIGHT, HEIGHT, AND HEAD CIRCUMFERENCE *(Continued)*

Age	Weight	Height	Head Circumference
12–18 mo (continued)	Average weight is 20–24 lb Birth weight is tripled by 12 mo		
18 mo–3 yr	Average weight is 28–30 lb Birth weight is quadrupled by 2 yr	Grows to 33–37 inches Approximately 50% of adult height by 2 yr	
3–6 yr	Average weight is 44 lb	Grows to 44 inches Birth length doubles by 4 yr Height and weight are even at 5 yr	
7–11 yr	Gains 5–7 lb per year	Growth appears in spurts Increases 3 inches per year to 52 inches at 7–10 yr	

NUTRITIONAL ASSESSMENT

Nutritional status affects the general health of a child and has a direct influence on a child's growth, development, cognition, and learning. A nutritional assessment is an essential component of a complete health history. A complete nutritional assessment incorporates information about dietary intake, clinical assessment of nutritional status, and biochemical status.

A thorough dietary history should be obtained by the nurse. The following types of questions should be included in your assessment:

- Usual mealtimes
- Which family member is responsible for meal preparation and shopping
- How much money is allotted for groceries each week
- How most foods are prepared (e.g., baked, fried, broiled, microwaved)
- How often the family eats out (frequency of fast food restaurants)
- Favorite foods, snacks
- Cultural practices or ethnic foods
- Food or beverage dislikes

Birth to 36 months: Girls
Length-for-age and Weight-for-age percentiles

NAME _____

RECORD # _____

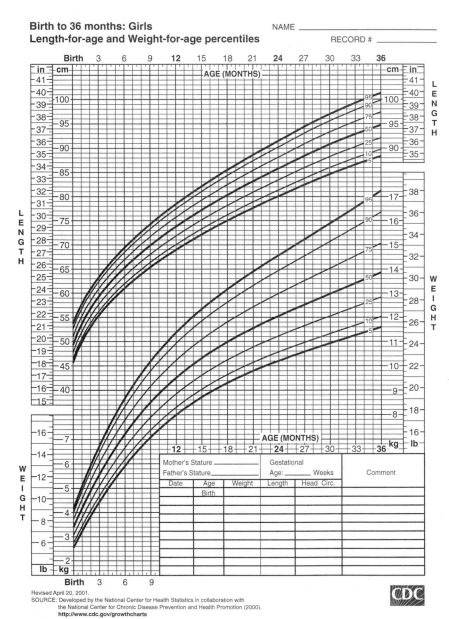

Revised April 20, 2001.
SOURCE: Developed by the National Center for Health Statistics in collaboration with
the National Center for Chronic Disease Prevention and Health Promotion (2000).
http://www.cdc.gov/growthcharts

A. Girls: Birth to 36 Months (Length and Weight)

Courtesy of National Center for Health Statistics, U.S. Centers for Disease Control and Prevention, 2001.

Birth to 36 months: Boys
Length-for-age and Weight-for-age percentiles

NAME _____

RECORD # _____

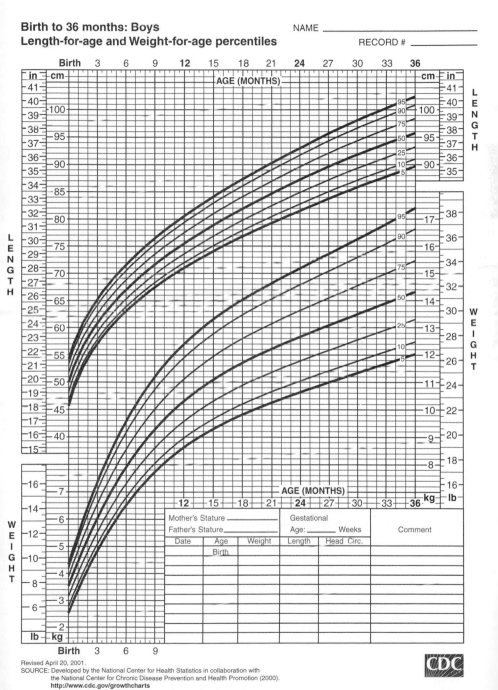

Revised April 20, 2001.
SOURCE: Developed by the National Center for Health Statistics in collaboration with
the National Center for Chronic Disease Prevention and Health Promotion (2000).
http://www.cdc.gov/growthcharts

B. Boys: Birth to 36 Months (Length and Weight)

**Birth to 36 months: Girls
Head circumference-for-age and
Weight-for-length percentiles**

NAME _____

RECORD # _____

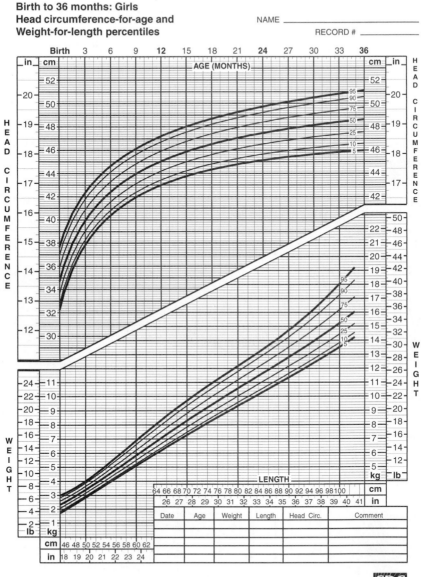

SOURCE: Developed by the National Center for Health Statistics in collaboration with
the National Center for Chronic Disease Prevention and Health Promotion (2000).
http://www.cdc.gov/growthcharts

C. Girls: Birth to 36 Months (Head Circumference)

Birth to 36 months: Boys
Head circumference-for-age and
Weight-for-length percentiles

NAME _____

RECORD # _____

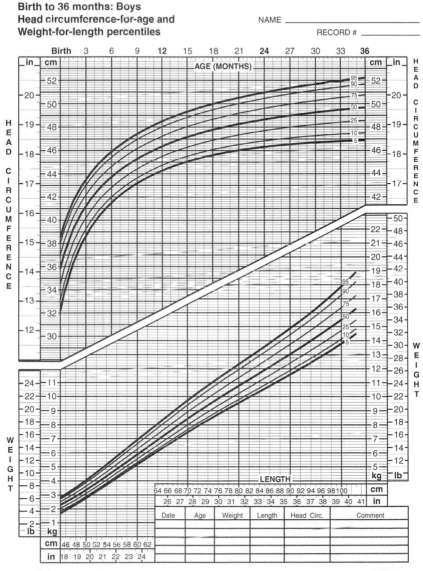

D. Boys: Birth to 36 Months (Head Circumference)

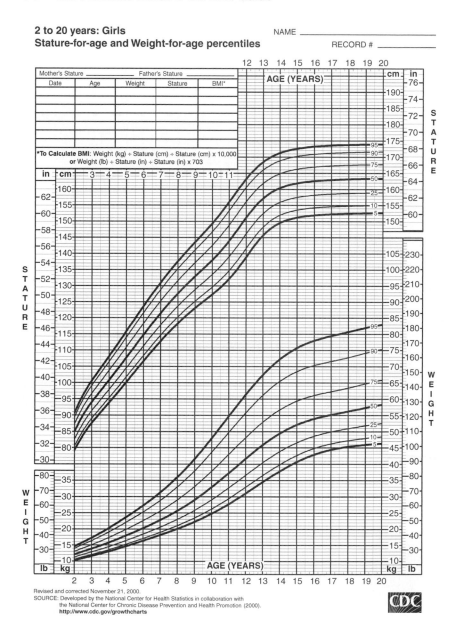

E. Girls: 2 to 20 Years (Stature and Weight)

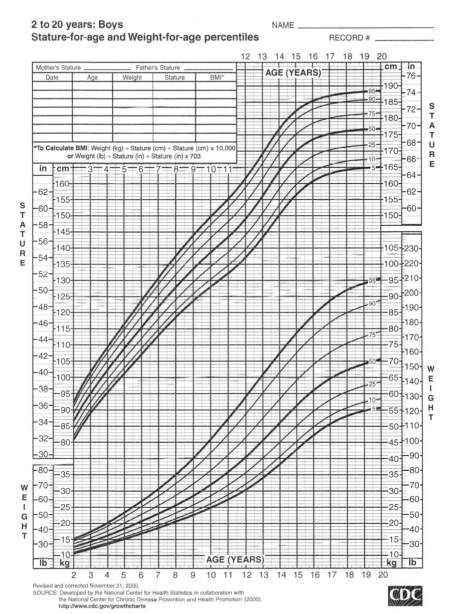

F. Boys: 2 to 20 Years (Stature and Weight)

- Description of child's usual appetite
- Feeding habits
- Breastfeeding
- Past medical history including any emotional difficulties
- Medication history
- Supplemental vitamins, herbs, iron, fluoride
- Food allergies
- Special diets
- Recent weight gain or loss
- Types of routine exercise

Additional information to obtain for young infants includes the following:

- Birth history (e.g., birth weight, history of prematurity, small for gestational age)
- Past medical history, especially in terms of gastrointestinal disturbances
- Feeding difficulties such as excessive fussiness, colic, regurgitation, difficulty swallowing and sucking

Dietary Intake

A thorough diet history should be obtained by the nurse. Food intake can be recorded by using a food diary or a food frequency record.

Record the following types of information in a food diary:

- Times of meals and snacks
- Description of food items including the actual food, amount, and method of preparation
- With whom the child ate
- Related factors such as associated activity, place, persons, feelings, hunger

Record the following types of information in a food frequency record:

- Food group (grains, vegetables, fruits, milk, meat and beans, fats, oils, and sweets)
- Numbers of servings per day or week in each of the food groups
- Serving size

The U.S. government released revised Dietary Guidelines for Americans in January 2005. The goal is to stop the dramatic and serious increase in obesity among U.S. children. Because of poor eating habits coupled with too little exercise, children are at substantial risk for major health problems such as diabetes and heart disease. The new food pyramid is now combined with suggestions for balancing food and physical activity. The specific suggestions (based upon a 2,000 cal/day diet) recommended by the U.S.

Department of Agriculture Center for Nutrition Policy and Promotion are summarized below:

- Grains—6 oz every day (3 of these should be whole grains)
- Vegetables—2½ cups every day (eat more green and orange vegetables; increase intake of dry beans and peas)
- Fruits—2 cups every day (variety is important; limit the amount of fruit juice)
- Milk—2 cups every day for children age 2 to 8 (for older children the amount should be increased to 3 cups per day; use low-fat or fat-free milk products)
- Meat and Beans—5½ oz per day (choose low-fat or lean meats and poultry; bake, broil, or grill; variety is important)
- Children and teenagers should be physically active for 60 minutes every day, or most days
- Most fat sources should be from fish, nuts, and vegetable oils; limit solid fats like butter, margarine, shortening, or lard; keep saturated fats, trans fats, and sodium intake low
- Food and beverages should be low in added sugars

Clinical Assessment

Another component of the nutritional assessment is the clinical examination of the child. This provides information regarding signs of adequate nutrition or deficiencies. Assessment of the skin, hair, mouth, teeth, eyes, neck, chest, abdomen, cardiovascular system, neurological system, and musculoskeletal system can be useful in determining possible nutritional deficits or excesses (see table on page 34 for physical signs of nutritional deficits). Anthropomorphic measurements of height, weight, head circumference, skinfold thickness, and arm circumference are also essential components of the physical examination.

Food Allergies

During the assessment of the child, it is essential to determine if the child has any history of food allergies. Although many children have food intolerances (i.e., skin rashes, GI upset), true food allergies trigger the immune system. Allergies can result in anaphylaxis, which can be fatal. Common food allergens include peanuts, eggs, tree nuts (e.g., pecans, walnuts), shellfish, milk, and soy. If a parent or child does report a history of food allergies, it is essential to obtain specific information about the type of food and type of reaction.

Food allergies are usually diagnosed by the child's pediatrician or pediatric allergist. Skin tests and blood tests (RAST testing) are performed.

PHYSICAL SIGNS ASSOCIATED WITH NUTRITIONAL DEFICITS

Body Part	Normal Appearance	Physical Signs	Nutritional Deficit or Excess
Skin	Uniform color, smooth, firm	Depigmentation, scaling, dry appearance, edema, pallor	Vitamin A, protein, riboflavin, vitamin B₁₂, excess sodium
Hair	Shiny, strong, not easily plucked	Dull, dry, thin, alopecia depigmentation	Protein, calories, vitamin C
Mouth	Lips smooth, pink, not chapped; tongue rough texture, no lesions; teeth white, no cavities; gums firm, pink; mucous membranes moist, pink, smooth	Lips reddened, swollen, cracked; tongue—glossitis; teeth brown, pitted, with caries; gums spongy, bleeding, swollen; mucous membranes with ulcers	Riboflavin, vitamin C, niacin, fluoride; excess carbohydrates, excess vitamin A
Eyes	Clear, bright, moist membranes	Pale conjunctiva, night blindness, corneal drying	Vitamin A, riboflavin
Neck	Thyroid not visible	Thyroid enlarged, grossly visible	Iodine
Chest	Chest is almost circular; lateral diameter increases in proportion to anteroposterior diameter in children	Depressed rib cage, protrusion of sternum	Vitamin D
Abdomen	Abdomen is slightly protruded; older children have flat abdomen	Abdominal distension, poor musculature	Protein, calories
Cardiovascular system	Heart rate and blood pressure within normal limits	Tachycardia, palpitations, arrhythmias, increased blood pressure	Potassium, magnesium; excess sodium
Neurological system	Alert, emotionally stable, intact reflexes	Irritable, listless, lethargic, diminished or absent deep tendon reflexes	Thiamin, niacin, vitamin C, vitamin E
Musculoskeletal system	Firm muscles, bilaterally equal strength, normal spinal curves, symmetric and straight extremities, full range of motion	Weak, wasting appearance; kyphosis, lordosis, or scoliosis, bowing of extremities	Protein, calories, vitamin D, calcium, vitamin A

Children who have documented food allergies will have been prescribed an EpiPen (containing epinephrine) which can be quickly given to stop an anaphylactic reaction. It is important to assess the caregiver and child's knowledge about using this device.

Biochemical Analysis

Biochemical analysis is the last integral component of the nutritional assessment. Blood chemistry levels of hematocrit and hemoglobin (indication of anemias), albumin (protein malnutrition), blood urea nitrogen (negative nitrogen balance), creatinine (high protein intake), lead (water consumption containing lead), glucose (dehydration, acidosis), and cholesterol (dietary-fat intake) should be analyzed. Normal values for these tests are located in Chapter 3.

CALCULATING DAILY CALORIC REQUIREMENTS

Body Weight (kg)	Caloric Expenditure/Day
Up to 10	100 kcal/kg
11–20	1,000 kcal + 50 kcal/kg for each kg above 10 kg
More than 20	1,500 kcal + 20 kcal/kg for each kg above 20 kg

These formulas are not appropriate for neonates less than 2 weeks old or for children with conditions associated with abnormal losses. In addition, children with disease, prior surgery, fever, or pain may require additional calories above the maintenance value. Children who are comatose or immobile may require fewer calories.

Breastfeeding

The numbers of mothers choosing to breastfeed have steadily increased over recent years. Breast milk has been shown to be the most beneficial food for a child. In fact, increasing the percentage of mothers who breastfeed their children has been identified as one of the Healthy People 2010 goals set by the U.S. Department of Health and Human Services. Breastfeeding is also recommended as the preferred method of feeding the child by the American Academy of Pediatrics (AAP) and the World Health Organization (WHO).

During hospitalization, mothers may have to express (or pump) their breast milk while the child is hospitalized. It is essential for the nurse to utilize basic knowledge regarding the safe storage of expressed human milk. These include the following:

- Milk can be stored at room temperature for up to 10 hours, in a refrigerator for up to 8 days, and inside a freezer for up to 3–4 months.

- Storage containers should be either hard plastic or glass with well-fitting tops or specially designed freezer milk bags designed for storing human milk.
- Storing milk in 2- to 4-oz servings may reduce waste.
- All expressed human milk should be labeled appropriately with the patient's name and the date of collection.
- Human milk can be thawed or heated under warm running water and should not be brought to a boiling point.
- Swirling of the milk before feeding will help to redistribute the cream into the milk as it is normal for stored milk to separate into a cream and milk layer.
- Thawed milk can be refrigerated for up to 24 hours. It should not be refrozen.
- Expressed milk can be kept in a common refrigerator. According to the U.S. Center for Disease Control and U.S. Occupational Safety and Health Administration, human milk is not among the body fluids that require special handling or storage in separate containers. Institutions should have established policies regarding the location to store human milk.

DEVELOPMENTAL ASSESSMENT

Children are at high risk for developmental delay and regression resulting from the stress of hospitalization. To most appropriately interact with children and to encourage their development, the nurse needs to be knowledgeable about normal growth and developmental milestones.

General Information

Patterns of development are sequential and predictable. Children must achieve one level before they can proceed to the next. Caregivers play an extremely important role in developmental assessment. Timing of speech and language development are most helpful in the determination of normalcy. Vision, hearing, and physical impairment, as well as illness and hospitalization, adversely affect the results of standardized developmental testing.

Developmental Characteristics

Infant (Birth to 1 year)—Erikson's Trust versus Mistrust

Personal or Social. Consistency of care is essential to the development of trust. Signaled needs must be met promptly and consistently.

Cognitive. The infant learns to separate self from other objects. The concept of object permanence, which develops at approximately 9 to 10 months, is necessary for the development of self-image.

Motor. The infant progresses from rolling over to reaching out to sitting to beginning to creep and crawl.

Toddler (1 to 3 years)—Erikson's Autonomy versus Shame and Doubt

Personal or Social. This is a period of holding on and letting go. Children begin to tolerate some separation from the parent. They engage in parallel play. Temper tantrums are an expression of frustration of not being able to verbalize wants. Children need rituals and a safe environment to develop autonomy. They use negativism in their quest for autonomy.

Language or Cognitive. The major achievement is language development. Appearance of an object denotes function. Children imitate household activities, and are very egocentric.

Motor. A major skill is the development of locomotion (e.g., walking, running, climbing). A major task is toilet training. Children develop a pincher grasp.

Preschooler (3 to 6 Years)—Erikson's Initiative versus Guilt

Personal or Social. Children need a security object. They are learning sex differences. They are energetic learners and feel guilt for not behaving or acting appropriately; they also may feel guilt from having thoughts that differ from the perceived norm. Beginnings of morality and the development of a conscience become evident. Children have a fear of mutilation and injury. They have poorly defined body boundaries and need a bandage to cover injuries to maintain body integrity.

Language or Cognitive. Preschoolers talk incessantly and in complete sentences. They have global organization of thought. Changing any part of something changes the whole thing. They give life-like qualities to inanimate objects. Preschoolers cannot perceive opposite behavior so caregivers need to phrase directions positively. They are shifting from total egocentricity to beginning to be able to consider other viewpoints. They have magical thinking and accept meaning literally.

Motor. Walking, running, climbing, and jumping are well established. Most children can use scissors by age 4 years and tie shoes by 5 years.

School-Age Child (6 to 12 years)—Erikson's Industry versus Inferiority

Personal or Social. The goal is to achieve a sense of personal and interpersonal competence by acquiring technologies and social skills. Failure to accomplish this leads to a sense of inferiority. Further development of conscience occurs. Peer groups are influential and necessary but caregivers are still the primary influence.

Language or Cognitive. Children use thought processes to explore events. They can see things from other points of view, and can reason. They are present-oriented and learn best with concrete examples.

Adolescent (12 to 18 years)—Erikson's Identity versus Role Confusion

Personal or Social. Adolescents are trying to develop a sense of identity. Early adolescents need peer approval; peer pressure may lead to risk-taking behaviors. Late adolescents need autonomy from their family and develop a sense of personal identity. They need a group identity to develop a personal identity. They are on an emotional roller coaster. Body image established during adolescence is retained throughout life.

Cognitive. Adolescents can think beyond the present and are concerned with the possible. Adolescents use logic and scientific reasoning, and are capable of abstract thinking. They want a clear picture of life and its purposes. They often believe they are invincible.

Developmental Assessment Tools

Optimum developmental screening should be done with healthy, nonhospitalized children. Children who are hospitalized may have multiple variables interfering with normal testing. There are many tools available. The most commonly used tool is the Denver II Developmental Screening Test. Although during hospitalization is not the optimum time to test children, this tool can be used as a quick reference for the sequencing of normal milestones and to help identify areas that would be appropriate for stimulation.

Denver II Developmental Screening Test

The Denver II is used to assess well children from birth to 6 years of age. It is designed to "compare a given child's performance on a variety of tasks to the performance of other children the same age" (Frankenburg & Dodds, 1990). It is not a predictor of future development and does not test intelligence quotient. To perform the Denver II, the nurse must be trained, must follow strict guidelines that are specific to testing and interpretation, and must use the kit with the materials provided. The Denver II assesses development in four general areas. The Denver II test follows, concluding with a summary of milestones assessed on the Denver II to assist the nurse in assessing and encouraging normal development in hospitalized children.

Revised Prescreening Developmental Questionnaire

The revised prescreening developmental questionnaire (R-PDQ) is a parent-answered prescreening questionnaire based on questions from the Denver II. It is used to assess children from birth to 6 years of age; four different forms are available based on age. This questionnaire gives the caregiver's perspective of the child's developmental abilities.

(Both of the aforementioned tests, with forms and complete instructions, are available from Denver Developmental Materials, Inc., P.O. Box 371075, Denver, CO 80237-5075; phone 800-419-4729.)

PAIN ASSESSMENT

Factors That Affect Children's Response to Pain

Culture
Developmental level
Caregiver attitudes
Expectations
Education or teaching
Type of anesthetic or procedure
Previous experience with pain
Caregiver's presence or absence
Nurse's or doctor's attitudes and beliefs about pain
Fear

Possible Physical Signs and Symptoms of Pain

Facial expression of discomfort, grimacing, or crying
Immobility or guarding area of body
Elevated pulse or respirations
Irritability or restlessness
Decreased appetite
Crying

Developmental Responses to Pain

Infants. Irritability, crying, withdrawal, pushing away, restless sleeping, poor feeding.

Toddlers. Very quiet, regressive behavior, uncooperative, crying, pointing to where it hurts (more accurate in pointing to where it hurts than saying where it hurts), say "ooww," fear responses. (May leave room to go to safe area of the playroom even though he or she hurts because the fear of what will happen in the room overshadows the pain.)

Preschoolers. Become quiet, may feel pain is punishment for bad behavior or thoughts. Good at procrastination before painful procedures

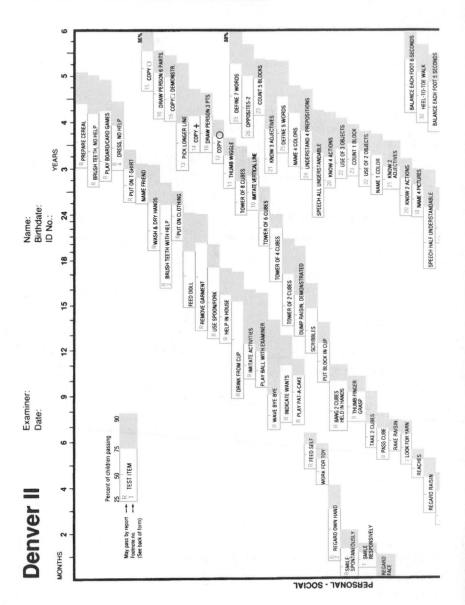

Denver II

Name:
Birthdate:
ID No.:

Examiner:
Date:

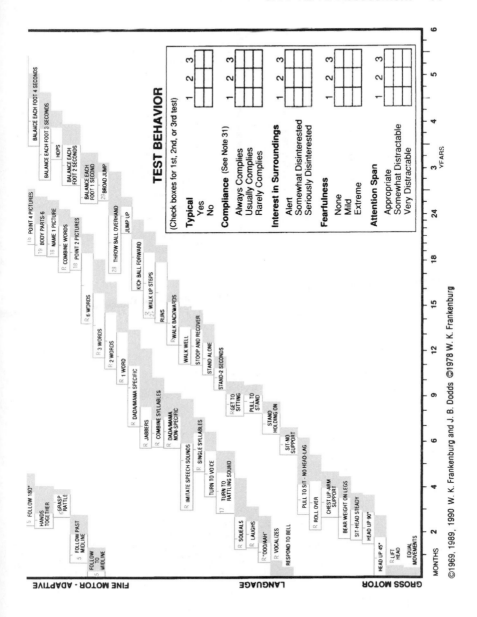

DIRECTIONS FOR ADMINISTRATION

1. Try to get child to smile by smiling, talking or waving. Do not touch him/her.
2. Child must stare at hand several seconds.
3. Parent may help guide toothbrush and put toothpaste on brush.
4. Child does not have to be able to tie shoes or button/zip in the back.
5. Move yarn slowly in an arc from one side to the other, about 8" above child's face.
6. Pass if child grasps rattle when it is touched to the backs or tips of fingers.
7. Pass if child tries to see where yarn went. Yarn should be dropped quickly from sight from tester's hand without arm movement.
8. Child must transfer cube from hand to hand without help of body, mouth, or table.
9. Pass if child picks up raisin with any part of thumb and finger.
10. Line can vary only 30 degrees or less from tester's line.
11. Make a fist with thumb pointing upward and wiggle only the thumb. Pass if child imitates and does not move any fingers other than the thumb.

12. Pass any enclosed form. Fail continuous round motions.

13. Which line is longer? (Not bigger.) Turn paper upside down and repeat. (pass 3 of 3 or 5 of 6)

14. Pass any lines crossing near midpoint.

15. Have child copy first. If failed, demonstrate.

When giving items 12, 14, and 15, do not name the forms. Do not demonstrate 12 and 14.

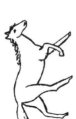

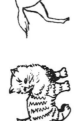

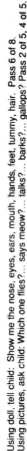

16. When scoring, each pair (2 arms, 2 legs, etc.) counts as one part.

17. Place one cube in cup and shake gently near child's ear, but out of sight. Repeat for other ear.

18. Point to picture and have child name it. (No credit is given for sounds only.)
    If less than 4 pictures are named correctly, have child point to picture as each is named by tester.

19. Using doll, tell child: Show me the nose, eyes, ears, mouth, hands, feet, tummy, hair. Pass 6 of 8.

20. Using pictures, ask child: Which one flies?... says meow?... talks?... barks?... gallops? Pass 2 of 5, 4 of 5.

21. Ask child: What do you do when you are cold?... tired?... hungry? Pass 2 of 3, 3 of 3.

22. Ask child: What do you do with a cup? What is a chair used for? What is a pencil used for?
    Action words must be included in answers.

23. Pass if child correctly places **and** says how many blocks are on paper. (1, 5).

24. Tell child: Put block **on** table; **under** table; **in front of** me, **behind** me. Pass 4 of 4.
    (Do not help child by pointing, moving head or eyes).

25. Ask child: What is a ball?... lake?... desk?... house?... banana?... curtain?... fence?... ceiling? Pass if defined in terms
    of use, shape, what it is made of, or general category (such as banana is fruit, not just yellow). Pass 5 of 8, 7 of 8.

26. Ask child: If a horse is big, a mouse is __? If fire is hot, ice is __? If the sun shines during the day, the moon shines
    during the __? Pass 2 of 3.

27. Child may use wall or rail only, not person. May not crawl.

28. Child must throw ball overhand 3 feet to within arm's reach of tester.

29. Child must perform standing broad jump over width of test sheet (8 1/2 inches).

30. Tell child to walk forward, 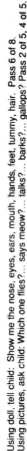 heel within 1 inch of toe. Tester may demonstrate.
    Child must walk 4 consecutive steps.

31. In the second year, half of normal children are non-compliant.

OBSERVATIONS:

DEVELOPMENTAL GUIDELINES: DENVER II

Age	Personal or Social	Fine Motor or Adaptive	Language	Gross Motor
Birth	Regards face	—	Vocalizes; responds to bell	Lifts head, equal movements
2 mo	Spontaneous and responsive smile	Follows person or object to midline	Makes ooh and ah sounds	Lifts head 30–45 degrees
4 mo	Looks at hand	Grasps rattle; holds hands together	Laughs; squeals	Lifts head up 90 degrees; sits with head steady; begins to bear weight
6 mo	Works for toy	Follows person or object 180 degrees; looks at small objects; reaches	Turns toward rattling sound	Chest up, arms supportive; rolls over; pulls to sit; no head lag
9 mo	Feeds self	Develops object permanence; passes block from hand to hand; holds block in each hand	Turns toward voice; uses single syllables; imitates sounds "Dada/Mama" nonspecific	Sits with no support; stands holding on to support
12 mo	Plays pat-a-cake; indicates wants; waves bye-bye	Develops thumb-finger grasp; bangs two objects together	Combines syllables; jabbers	Pulls to stand; gets to sitting; stands 2 sec
15 mo	Begins to play ball; imitates activities; drinks from cup	Puts objects in cup	"Dada/Mama" specific plus knows one to two words	Stands alone; stoops, recovers; walks well
18 mo	Can use spoon	Scribbles; dumps things; builds a tower of two blocks	Knows two to six words	Walks backward; runs
2 yr	Removes own clothes	Builds a tower of two to four blocks	Knows six or more words; combines words	Runs well; walks up steps; kicks ball
3 yr	Puts on own clothes; washes and dries hands; brushes teeth with help	Builds a tower of six blocks	Knows six body parts; speech half understandable	Throws ball overhand; jumps up
4 yr	Puts on T-shirt	Builds tower of eight blocks; imitates vertical line; wiggles thumb	Names one color; counts 1 block; speech all understandable	Can do broad jump; balances for 2 sec on each foot
5 yr	Gets dressed without help	Draws three-part person; copies a "+"	Names four colors; understands "on," "under," "in front of," "behind"	Hops; balances for 3–4 sec on each foot
6 yr	Prepares cereal; brushes teeth with no help	Draws six-part person; copies a square; picks larger line	Knows cold, tired, hungry; counts five blocks; knows opposites	Walks heel-to-toe; balances for 6 sec on each foot

44

(persistent "Wait a minute" or "I have to go to the bathroom"). May be able to tell where it hurts and use tools to describe the severity.

School-Age Children. May deny pain to be brave or to avoid further hurt. May withdraw, or watch or stare at the television.

Adolescents. Fear loss of control. Are affected by mood changes and expectations of behavior. May refuse or overrequest medication. Show increased muscle tension.

Assessment Guidelines

Assess frequently and uniformly using age-appropriate tools and nursing observations. Tools help to more accurately assess and record pain assessment and need to be used and recorded at least once a shift and 30 minutes to an hour after the pain-relief method is applied or pain medication is given. This provides a record to determine whether pain is increasing or decreasing and whether relief methods are effective.

Consult hospital or institutional policy regarding tools used in your facility and read original information and guidelines for their use.

Pain Assessment Tools

FLACC Behavioral Pain Scale.

FLACC BEHAVIORAL PAIN SCALE

Categories	Score 0	Score 1	Score 2
Face	No particular expression or smile	Occasional grimace or frown, withdrawn, disinterested	Frequent to constant frown, clenched jaw, quivering chin
Legs	Normal position or relaxed	Uneasy, restless, tense	Kicking, or legs drawn up
Activity	Lying quietly, normal position, moves easily	Squirming, shifting back and forth, tense	Arched, rigid, or jerking
Cry	No cry (awake or asleep)	Moans or whimpers, occasional complaint	Crying steadily, screams or sobs, frequent complaints
Consolability	Content, relaxed	Reassured by occasional touching, hugging, or being talked to, distractable	Difficult to console or comfort

---

Merkel, S., Voepel-Lewis, T., Shayevitz, J., & Malviya, S. (1997). The FLACC: A behavioral scale for scoring postoperative pain in young children. *Pediatric Nursing, 23*(3), 293–297.

Clients who are awake: Observe for at least 2–5 minutes. Observe legs and body uncovered. Reposition client or observe activity, and assess body for tenseness and tone. Initiate consoling interventions if needed.

Clients who are asleep: Observe for at least 5 minutes or longer. Observe body and legs uncovered. If possible, reposition the client. Touch the body and assess for tenseness and tone.

Face: Score 0 points if client has a relaxed face, eye contact, and interest in surroundings. Score 1 point if client has a worried look to face, with eyebrows lowered, eyes partially closed, cheeks raised, or mouth pursed. Score 2 points if client has deep furrows in the forehead, with closed eyes, open mouth, and deep lines around nose and lips.

Legs: Score 0 points if client has usual tone and motion to limbs (legs and arms). Score 1 point if client has increased tone, rigidity, is tense, or has intermittent flexion or extension of limbs. Score 2 points if client has hypertonicity, legs pulled tight, exaggerated flexion or extension of limbs, or tremors.

Activity: Score 0 points if client moves easily and freely, with normal activity or restrictions. Score 1 point if client shifts positions, is hesitant to move, or has guarding, tense torso, or pressure on body part. Score 2 points if the client is in a fixed position, rocking, has side-to-side head movement, and is rubbing a body part.

Cry: Score 0 points if client has no cry or moan when awake or asleep. Score 1 point if client has occasional moans, cries, whimpers, or sighs. Score 2 points if client has frequent or continuous moans, cries, or grunts.

Consolability: Score 0 points if client is calm and does not require consoling. Score 1 point if client responds to comfort by touch or talk in 1/2–1 minute. Score 2 points if client requires constant comforting or is unable to be consoled.

Whenever feasible, behavioral measurement of pain should be used in conjunction with self-report. When self-report is not possible, interpretation of pain behaviors and decision making regarding treatment of pain requires careful consideration of the context in which the pain behaviors were observed.

Each category is scored on the 0–2 scale, which results in a total score of 0–10. **Assessment of Behavioral Score:** 0 = Relaxed and comfortable. 1–3 = Mild discomfort. 4–6 = Moderate pain. 7–10 = Severe discomfort or pain.

Numeric Scale. The numeric scale rates pain from 0 to 10, where 0 is no hurt, and 10 is the worst hurt ever experienced. Child picks a number between 0 and 10 to describe the severity of hurt. The child must know numbers; this works best with children ages 5 years and older.

Poker Chip Tool. This tool uses five poker chips to measure pieces of hurt. It works best with children ages 4 and older.

Color Tool. This tool uses an outline of the body. The child chooses a color to indicate the degree of hurt and colors where it hurts.

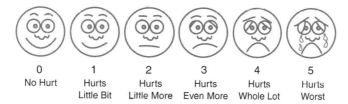

0	1	2	3	4	5
No Hurt	Hurts Little Bit	Hurts Little More	Hurts Even More	Hurts Whole Lot	Hurts Worst

Explain to the person that each face is for a person who feels happy because he has no pain (hurt) or sad because he has some or a lot of pain. Face 0 is very happy because he doesn't hurt at all. Face 1 hurts just a little bit. Face 2 hurts a little more. Face 3 hurts even more. Face 4 hurts a whole lot. Face 5 hurts as much as you can imagine, although you don't have to be crying to feel this bad. Ask the person to choose the face that best describes how he is feeling.

Rating scale is recommended for persons age 3 years and older.

From Hockenberry M.J., Wilson D., Winkelstein M.L.: *Wong's Essentials of Pediatric Nursing*, ed. 7, St. Louis, 2005, p. 1259. Used with permission. Copyright Mosby.

Wong-Baker FACES Pain Scale.
This pain assessment tool can be used with children as young as age 3.

ASSESSMENT AND CARE OF THE POSTOPERATIVE CLIENT

Prepare the client's room for his or her return by turning bed down and ensuring that any pumps or suction equipment, emesis basin, or other needed equipment is ready.

Receive the client from recovery room.

Review orders, operative note, and PACU report.

Check vital signs immediately and as ordered, usually at least every 4 hours.

Assess skin color and turgor.

Assess level of consciousness.

Assess for pain routinely; document assessment and medicate as needed.

Check dressing and reinforce as needed; mark outline of discharge or bleeding on dressing.

Assess for bleeding elsewhere.

Check for bowel sounds.

Assess for bladder distension.

Keep accurate record of intake and output.

Encourage the client to turn, cough, and breathe deeply as condition permits. Encourage use of incentive spirometer.

Splint incision before encouraging coughing.
Report any excessive bleeding or abnormal vital signs.

ASSESSING LEVEL OF CONSCIOUSNESS IN CHILDREN

The Glasgow Coma Scale (GCS) is a standardized, objective assessment tool used to assess level of consciousness (LOC) in children. Nurses use their observational skills in three areas: eye opening, verbal response, and motor response. A value of 1 to 5 is assigned to each of the three areas. The sum of these numerical values is the objective measurement used to report LOC. A child with a score of 15 (highest) represents unaltered LOC. The lowest score of 3 represents deep coma or death. A score of 8 or less generally represents a comatose state. The pediatric version of the GCS recognizes the developmental variations among children of different ages in relation to expected verbal and motor responses.

MODIFIED PEDIATRIC GLASGOW COMA SCALE

		Score	
Eye opening	Spontaneously	4	
	To speech	3	
	To pain	2	
	None	1	
Best motor	Obeys commands	6	
response	Localizes pain	5	
(usually record	Flexion withdrawal	4	
best arm or	Flexion abnormal	3	
age-appropriate	Extension	2	
response)	None	1	

	Younger than 2 yr		Older than 2 yr
Best response	Oriented	5	Smiles, listens, follows
to auditory or	Confused	4	Cries, consolable
visual stimulus	Inappropriate words	3	Inappropriate persistent cry
	Incomprehensible words	2	Agitated, restless
	None	1	None
	Endotracheal tube	T	
	Coma Scale Total	_____	

ASSESSMENT AND CARE OF THE ORTHOPEDIC CLIENT

Cast Care

Remember that Plaster-of-Paris casts can take from 10 to 72 hours to dry completely.

Remember that fiberglass and other synthetic materials dry within 30 minutes.

Expose cast to air until dry.

Handle a wet cast with palms of hands to prevent denting it with the fingers.

Check movement, sensation, pulses, and capillary refill of distal digits and compare bilaterally.

Elevate casted extremity to decrease swelling.

Keep small items that could be placed in the cast away from small children.

Use ice packs to help with itching and swelling.

Assess and medicate for pain as needed.

Traction Care

Assess alignment and pull.

Assess skin integrity under bandages for skin traction; change as needed when permitted.

Check pin sites in skeletal traction frequently for infection and bleeding. Clean and dress as ordered.

Assess neurovascular status as described in the physical examination section of this text.

Make sure ropes and pulleys are in original position and in good condition.

Keep bed in position ordered for desired pull.

Ensure ordered weight and keep weights hanging freely and out of traffic paths.

Provide pressure-reducing mattress.

Assess for skin breakdown in pressure areas.

Assess and medicate for pain as needed.

ASSESSMENT OF SEXUAL MATURATION

The predictable development of secondary sexual characteristics during puberty is divided into five phases termed *Tanner stages*. Although the order of this development is predictable, the ages at which these changes occur varies.

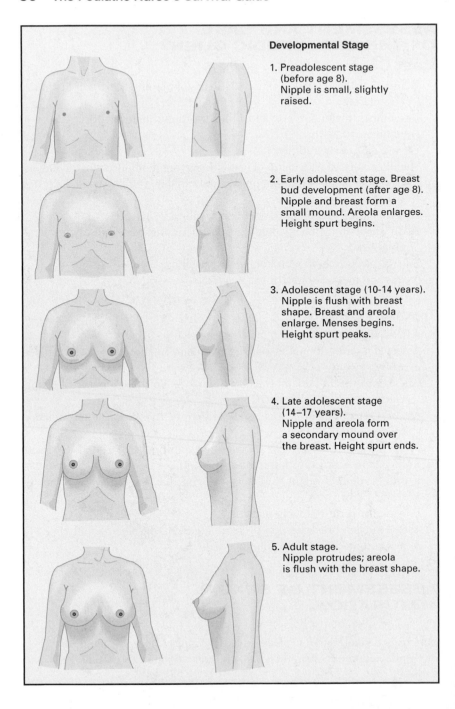

Developmental Stage

1. Preadolescent stage (before age 8). Nipple is small, slightly raised.

2. Early adolescent stage. Breast bud development (after age 8). Nipple and breast form a small mound. Areola enlarges. Height spurt begins.

3. Adolescent stage (10-14 years). Nipple is flush with breast shape. Breast and areola enlarge. Menses begins. Height spurt peaks.

4. Late adolescent stage (14–17 years). Nipple and areola form a secondary mound over the breast. Height spurt ends.

5. Adult stage. Nipple protrudes; areola is flush with the breast shape.

Stage 1

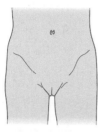

Preadolescent Stage
(before age 8)
No pubic hair, only body hair (vellus hair)

Stage 4

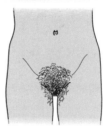

Late Adolescent Stage
(ages 13 to 15)
Texture and curl of pubic hair is similar to that of an adult but not spread to thighs

Stage 2

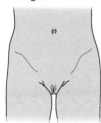

Early Adolescent Stage
(ages 8 to 12)
Sparse growth of long, slightly dark, fine pubic hair, slightly curly and located along the labia

Stage 5

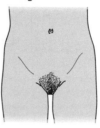

Adult Stage
Adult appearance in quality and quantity of pubic hair; growth is spread to inner aspect of thighs and abdomen

Stage 3

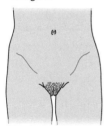

Adolescent Stage
(ages 12 to 13)
Pubic hair becomes darker, curlier, and spreads over the symphysis

Sexual Maturity in Females

Externally examine the female for secondary sexual characteristic development. Specifically, growth of breast tissue and pubic hair are assessed. The onset of breast development and pubic hair growth occurs between the ages of 8½ to 13. The progression between stages 2 and 5 usually takes an average of 3 years. Menarche usually occurs during breast stage 3 or 4.

	Pubic Hair	**Penis**	**Testes**
1.	No pubic hair, only fine body hair (vellus hair)	Preadolescent; childhood size and proportion	Preadolescent; childhood size and proportion
2.	Sparse growth of long, slightly dark, straight hair	Slight or no growth	Growth in testes and scrotum; scrotum reddens and changes texture
3.	Becomes darker and coarser; slightly curled and spreads over symphysis	Growth, especially in length	Further growth
4.	Texture and curl of pubic hair is similar to that of an adult but not spread to thighs	Further growth in length; diameter increases; development of glans	Further growth; scrotum darkens
5.	Adult appearance in quality and quantity of pubic hair; growth is spread to medial surface of thighs	Adult size and shape	Adult size and shape

Sexual Maturity in Males

Externally examine the male for secondary sexual characteristic development. Specifically, growth of the testes and penis are assessed. The first changes in males are testicular enlargement with corresponding thinning, reddening, and loosening of the scrotum. This usually begins between ages $9\frac{1}{2}$ to $13\frac{1}{2}$. Maturation from preadolescent to adult usually occurs over a 3-year period.

ASSESSMENT FOR CHILD ABUSE

Failure to Thrive (nonorganic)

Lack of normal growth and development

Usually affects those 18 months and younger

Weight is below the 5th percentile

Language delay

Is irritable, resists cuddling, and is unresponsive to nurturing

Appears thin, frail, undernourished

Has big, vacant eyes

May have gaze aversion

Has drawn, pinched, anxious or expressionless face; usually will not smile

Is obsessed with thumb or pacifier

Usually gains weight in hospital on same formula that he or she was on at home

Physical Abuse

Physical abuse is characterized by certain types of behaviors and injuries. The prevalent types of child abuse are physical abuse, sexual abuse, emotional abuse, and child neglect. Actually, neglect is the most common form of abuse. Regretfully, abuse cases are speculated to be drastically underreported. One of the major roles of the pediatric nurse is identification of abusive situations. Nurses (and other health care providers) must adhere to mandated reporting laws. Directions for reporting abuse vary from state to state and nurses must be familiar with procedures specific to the state in which they practice. Confidentiality is waived in child abuse situations. State reporting statutes include provisions that protect the nurse from legal liability as long as the reporting was conducted in good faith. Additionally, in many states, nurses may be subject to legal action (both civil and criminal) if they fail to report suspected abuse to the appropriate authorities.

Behaviors Suspicious of Abuse

The following are characteristic behaviors typical of a child who is abused:

Withdrawn

Does not cry or respond to painful procedures

May accuse adult
May try to console the caregiver

Some characteristic behaviors of the caregiver of an abused child are as follows:

Delays seeking treatment
Is unable to comfort child
Decreases number of visits
Uses multiple different health providers
Lacks follow-through
Blames child or child's sibling

In addition, there may be a variation in the child's history, the injury does not fit the history, and the accused caregiver is absent from visits.

Injuries Suspicious of Abuse

Bruises over soft tissue areas
Multiple planes of bruises
Multiple ages of bruises
    Approximate dating of bruises (related to hemoglobin breakdown)

0–2 days	swollen and tender
0–5 days	red-blue
5–7 days	greenish yellow
7–10 days	yellow to brown
10–14 days	brown
2–4 weeks	clear

Fractures of different ages
Bilateral black eyes including upper lids
Slap, grab marks
Human bite marks with greater than 3 cm between canines (consistent with adult teeth)
Linear bruises from belt
Bruises shaped like the object used to inflict them
Tie marks on extremities
Gag marks
Cigarette burns
Dry contact burns that are second degree
Forced immersion burns (dunking or donut burns)—the buttocks and feet are usually spared because they were held against the cool bottom of the tub; there are no splash marks; and there is a clear line of demarcation between burned and unburned areas of skin

Stocking or glove burns with no splash marks—usually are clearly demar-
  cated and go above the ankle or the wrist

Subdural hematomas with retinal hemorrhages from a shaking injury

Boggy scalp resulting from subgaleal hematomas caused by lifting the
  scalp off the skull

Traumatic alopecia or hair loss with tender scalp and broken hairs around
  patch of missing hair

Spiral fractures of the humerus or femur from a twisting injury

Any fracture in an infant

Bucket-handle fracture (chipped metaphysis) of femur or humerus, occur-
  ring because the child's ligaments are stronger than his or her bones

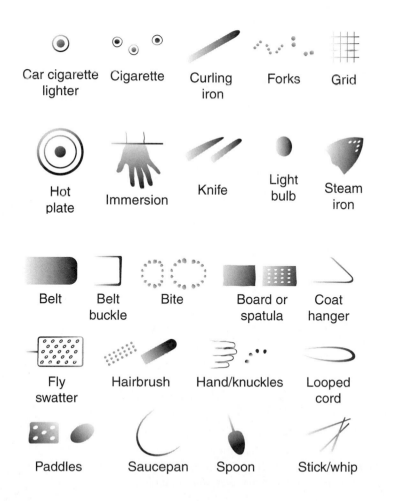

Signs of Sexual Abuse

Usually, few physical signs are present, but the following may be observed:

Abdominal or genital bruising
Lacerations of vagina or rectum
Sexually transmitted diseases in prepubertal child
Genital irritation or pain
Pregnancy

The following are behavioral signs typical of sexual abuse:

Advanced knowledge of explicit sexual behavior
Sexual acting out
Withdrawal
Fear of adult males or females
Depression
Encopresis (incontinence of stool)
Enuresis (incontinence of urine)
Runaway behaviors
Substance abuse

The child's story often is the only evidence of the abuse. The nurse must believe the child. Abused children need support and, most importantly, need to know that the abuse is not in any way their fault. The guilt is tremendous and they need praise for having the courage to tell.

Munchausen Syndrome by Proxy

Child is usually 6 years old or younger
Child's signs and symptoms cannot be explained by known disease etiologies
Tests, X-ray films, and studies are negative
Child has repeated hospitalizations for the same problem
Perpetrator is usually the mother
Mother's history is unsupported by other caregivers
Child improves when mother is not present
Possible positive family history, especially siblings with same problems
Mother is overinvolved and has some type of experience in health care
Father is absent or uninvolved

SIGNS AND SYMPTOMS OF ILLICIT DRUG EXPOSURE OR USE

Neonatal Exposure

Symmetrical growth retardation, decreased weight and FOC
Poor response to auditory and visual stimuli, may be sleepy or easily overstimulated and may become irritable

Poor feeding versus hyperphagia (rapidly sucks down 3 to 4 oz at first
feeding)
Vomiting or diarrhea
Sweating
Excessive crying, shrill cry or irritable
Jittery, has tremors
Hyperreflexia or increased muscle tone versus decreased muscle tone
Frantic hand sucking
Pallor
Poor sleeping
Frequent sneezing or yawning
Temperature instability
Seizure

Drug Use
Physical Signs and Symptoms (and Possible Drug Association)
Headache (inhalants)
Hyperreflexia (cocaine, hallucinogens)
Hyporeflexia (narcotics, heroin)
Slurred speech, ataxia (alcohol)
Bulky muscles (steroids)
Jaundice (alcohol)
Tachycardia, elevated blood pressure (alcohol, cocaine, hallucinogens)
Bradycardia, decreased blood pressure (heroin, narcotics)
Chest pain (cocaine)
Increased respirations (cocaine)
Decreased respirations (alcohol, heroin, narcotics)
Rhinorrhea (alcohol)
Erythematous nasal septum (cocaine, inhalants)
Epistaxis (cocaine)
Red, bloodshot eyes or conjunctivitis (alcohol, marijuana, inhalants)
Dilated pupils (cocaine)
Constricted pupils (heroin, narcotics)
Needle marks (heroin, narcotics)
Rapid precipitous delivery in primipara (cocaine)
Social Signs and Symptoms
Multiple accidents
Multiple sexually transmitted diseases
Aggressive behavior
Antisocial behavior

Psychologic Signs and Symptoms
Depression
Anxiety
Sleep changes
Hallucinations
Euphoria
Mood changes (excessive)
Memory loss or blackouts

CHAPTER 3

CLINICAL VALUES AND STANDARDS

CALCULATING DAILY MAINTENANCE FLUID REQUIREMENTS IN CHILDREN

Body weight (kg)	Amount of fluid per day
1–10 kg	100 mL/kg
11–20 kg	1,000 mL + 50 mL/kg for each kg more than 10 kg
>20 kg	1,500 mL + 20 mL/kg for each kg more than 20 kg

Urine output should average 0.5–1.0 mL/kg per hour when the child's fluid intake is adequate.

NORMAL LABORATORY VALUES AND INTERPRETATION

Acetaminophen

Therapeutic concentration	10–30 μg/mL
Toxic concentration	>200 μg/mL

Alanine Aminotransferase (ALT)/Serum Glutamic-Pyruvic Transaminase (SGPT)

Infant	<54 Units/L
Child or adult	1–30 Units/L

- Major sources: liver, skeletal muscle, and myocardium
- Increased in severe hepatitis, infectious mononucleosis, congestive heart failure (CHF), and eclampsia
- Not as specific for liver function as aspartate aminotransferase (AST)

Aldolase

Newborn	<32 Units/L
Child	<16 Units/L
Adult	<8 Units/L

- Major sources: skeletal muscle, myocardium, and liver
- Increased in muscular tissue damage and progressive muscular dystrophy
- Not increased in myasthenia gravis or multiple sclerosis

Alkaline Phosphatase

Infant	150–420 Units/L
2–10 yr	100–320 Units/L
11–18 yr (male)	100–390 Units/L
11–18 yr (female)	100–320 Units/L
Adult	30–120 Units/L

- Major sources: bone, intestinal mucosa, liver, placenta, and kidney
- Increase is normal in pregnancy
- Increased in biliary obstruction, bone metastasis or destruction, and malignant liver tumors

Benign transient hyperphosphatemia can occur in young children for 4–8 weeks.

Amylase

Newborn	0–44 Units/L
Adult	0–88 Units/L

- Major sources: pancreas, salivary glands, and ovaries
- Most common reason for increase is pancreatitis
- Levels are high in alcoholism, pregnancy, and diabetic ketoacidosis with a salivary origin

Antinuclear Antibodies (ANAs)

Not significant	<1:80
Likely significant	>1:320

- Used to rule out systemic lupus erythematosus (SLE), but can also be increased in rheumatoid arthritis (RA), scleroderma, carcinoma, tuberculosis (TB), and hepatitis

Antistreptolysin-O (ASO) Titer

Preschool	<1:85
School age	<1:170
Older adult	<1:85

- A 4x rise in paired serial specimens is significant
- Antibodies appear 7–10 days after acute streptococcal infection
- Also can be increased in liver disease

Aspartate Aminotransferase (AST)/Serum Glutamic-Oxaloacetic Transaminase (SGOT)

Newborn or infant 20–65 Units/L
Child or adult   0–35 Units/L

- Major sources: liver, skeletal muscle, kidney, myocardium, and erythrocytes
- Increased in liver necrosis, Reye's syndrome, hepatitis, myocardial infarction (MI), and infectious mononucleosis
- Not likely to be decreased

Bicarbonate (HCO₃)

Infant   20–24 mEq/L
>2 years   22–26 mEq/L

- Functions as a buffer to keep pH normal
- Increased in metabolic alkalosis
- Decreased in metabolic acidosis

Bilirubin (Total)

Term infants
 Cord   <2 mg/dL
 0–1 day <6 mg/dL
 1–2 days <8 mg/dL
 3–7 days <12 mg/dL
>1 month 0.2–1 mg/dL
Adult   0.1–1 mg/dL

Direct (Bili conjugated [BC])

0–0.4 mg/dL

BC is increased in conditions that cause obstruction in normal bile flow.

Indirect (Bili unconjugated [BU])

Total − direct = indirect
(Total − BC = BU)

BU is increased in any condition that causes hemolysis of red blood cells (RBCs).

Blood Urea Nitrogen (BUN)

5–25 mg/dL

- Used primarily to assess renal function but is affected by protein breakdown, hydration, and liver failure

- Increased in severe dehydration and impaired renal perfusion
- Decreased in overhydration

Calcium-Total Serum (Ca)

<1 week	7–12 mg/dL
Child	8–10.5 mg/dL
Adult	8.5–10.5 mg/dL

- Increased in dehydration, vitamin D intoxication, and metastatic bone disease
- Decreased in chronic renal disease, severe malnutrition, and low albumin levels

Carbon Dioxide Content (CO$_2$)

Infant or child	20–24 mEq/L
Adult	24–30 mEq/L

- Is an indirect measure of serum bicarbonate and is usually 2 mEq/L greater than the actual bicarbonate level
- Changes signify changes in acid-base balance

Chloride (Cl)

94–106 mEq/L

- Increases as sodium increases
- Decreases commonly caused by loss from vomiting, diarrhea, and diuretics

Cholesterol

Infant	53–135 mg/dL
Child	70–175 mg/dL
Adolescent	120–210 mg/dL
Adult	140–250 mg/dL

>35 mg/dL (high-density lipoprotein) "good cholesterol"
<110 mg/dL (low-density lipoprotein) "bad cholesterol"

- Increased in those with diets high in cholesterol and saturated fats
- Some also have genetic predispositions
- Decreased in hyperthyroidism, severe liver damage, and malnutrition

Complete Blood Count (CBC)

RBCs (Erythrocyte count)

Newborn	5.5–6 million/mm^3
Child	4.6–4.8 million/mm^3

Adult (male)   4.6–5.9 million/mm^3
     (female)   4.2–5.4 million/mm^3

- Increased number in high altitudes, increased physical strain, chronic lung disease, and cyanotic heart disease
- Decreased because of abnormal loss or destruction and bone marrow suppression

Descriptors of RBCs
Hypochromic—less color
Normochromic—normal color
Microcytic—small size
Normocytic—normal size
Macrocytic—large size

Hemoglobin (Hgb, Hb)
Newborn   17–19 g
Child   14 17 g
Adult (male)   13–18 g
     (female)   12–16 g

- If increased, look at in relation to the number and size of RBCs
- Decreased in all conditions that cause a decrease in RBCs (e.g., abnormal [Hgb], increased fragility leading to increased destruction)

Hematocrit (Hct)
Newborn   up to 65%
Child (mean)
     2 wks   53%
     1 mo   44%
     2 mo   35%
     6 mo–2 yr   36%
     2–6 yr   37%
     6–12 yr   40%
     12–18 yr (male)   43%
          (female)   41%
Adult (male)   45%–52%
     (female)   37%–48%

- Is the packed cell volume or the percentage of RBCs in plasma
- Is roughly three times the Hgb
- Capillary values may be 5%–10% higher than vena puncture
- Increase in normally hydrated child indicates a true increase in RBCs
- Can be increased in dehydration and decreased in overhydration

Mean corpuscular volume (MCV)

Newborn   95–121 μm^3
6–24 mo   70–86 μm^3
   Gradually increases to 78–98 μm^3
   Describes the average RBC volume

$$Hct \div RBC = MCV$$

- If less than 86 μm^3, the RBCs are considered microcytic and possibly indicates iron-deficiency anemia, lead poisoning, or thalassemia
- If greater than 98 μm^3, the RBCs are considered macrocytic and indicates possible pernicious anemia or folic-acid deficiency

Mean corpuscular hemoglobin (MCH)

27–32 pg

- Amount of Hgb in a single cell

$$(Hgb \times 10)/RBC = MCH$$

Mean corpuscular hemoglobin concentration (MCHC)

32%–36%

- Proportion of each cell occupied by Hgb
- Increased in congenital spherocytosis
- May be increased in normal newborns and sickle cell disease
- Decreased in microcytic anemias including iron-deficiency anemia

RBC Distribution Width (RDW)

11.5%–14.5%

- Variation of cell width
- May help assess types of anemias
- Iron-deficiency anemia increases the RDW; thalassemia does not
- Also increased in anisocytosis, reticulocytosis, and hemolysis, as well as in newborns

Platelets (Plt)

Newborn   100,000–290,000/mm^3
Child   150,000–350,000/mm^3
Adult   150,000–350,000/mm^3

- Have an 8- to 10-day life span
- Aid in coagulation by adhering and clumping to the wall of the vessel
- Increased (thrombocytosis) in malignancy and polycythemia
- Decreased (thrombocytopenia) in idiopathic thrombocytopenic purpura (ITP), after viral illness, in AIDS, in bone marrow suppression, and in patients with enlarged spleens, which destroy them too quickly

White blood cells (WBCs)

Newborn	10,000–35,000
Child	8,000–14,500
Adult	4,300–10,000

- Total WBC count
- Increased in bacterial infection and leukemias, especially acute lymphocytic leukemia
- Decreased in bone marrow suppression, in overwhelming sepsis, and with certain types of chemotherapy

Differential (diff) (mean %)

Neutrophils (segs)	54–62%
Bands	3–5%
Lymphocytes	25–33%
Monocytes	3–7%
Eosinophils	1–3%
Basophils	0–0.75%

- Total percentage must add up to 100%
- Left shift is usually seen in bacterial infections
- The left side of the diff (neutrophils and bands) increases
- Left shift also may be calculated as an immature to total (IT) neutrophil ratio of 0.20 or greater:

  IT = bands (immature) ÷ bands and neutrophils (total) ≥ 0.20

Absolute neutrophil count (ANC) = % of neutrophils + % of bands × number of WBCs

  Example: WBC count = 10,000, neutrophils = 51% bands = 2%

  51% + 2% = 53% 10,000 = ANC of 5,300

Neutropenia is an ANC < 1,500

- Segs: segmented neutrophils, mature form
- Bands: immature form of neutrophil
  - Are increased in bacterial infections, inflammatory processes, and tissue necrosis
  - Are decreased (neutropenia) in viral diseases, hepatitis, influenza, measles, mumps, rubella, and overwhelming infections
- Lymph: lymphocytes:
  - Principal component of the immune system:
    T lymphocyte is approximately 60%–80%
    B lymphocyte is approximately 5%–15%
    Non-T, non-B lymphocyte is approximately 10%–20%
  - Are increased in viral infections, mumps, hepatitis, retrovirus, infectious mononucleosis, tumors, and TB
  - Significantly increased in lymphocytic leukemias
  - Decreased in AIDS, severe malnutrition, and any condition that increases the neutrophils
- Mono: monocytes
  - Increase usually results from chronic conditions such as TB, malaria, and Rocky Mountain spotted fever
- Baso: basophils
  - Increased in malignancy
- Eos: eosinophils
  - Increased in allergic reactions, asthma, drug reactions, and parasitic infections
  - Decreased in corticosteroid use

Creatinine (Serum)

Newborn	0.3–1 mg/dL
Infant	0.2–0.4 mg/dL
Child	0.3–0.7 mg/dL
Adolescent	0.5–1 mg/dL
Adult (male)	0.6–1.3 mg/dL
(female)	0.5–1.2 mg/dL

- Used only to evaluate renal function
- Does not increase until at least half the nephrons are nonfunctioning

Erythrocyte Sedimentation Rate (ESR)

Newborn	0–4 mm/hr
Child	4–20 mm/hr
Adult (male)	0–20 mm/hr
(female)	0–10 mm/hr

- Normally increased during pregnancy
- Increase usually results from inflammation or tissue injury
- >100 mm/hr usually is a result of infection, malignant tumors, or collagen diseases
- Often used to monitor the course of RA, pelvic inflammatory disease, or infectious states in persons with AIDS

Ferritin

Newborn	25–200 ng/mL
1 mo	200–600 ng/mL
6 mo	50–200 ng/mL
6 mo–15 yr	7–140 ng/mL
Adult (male)	15–200 ng/mL
(female)	12–150 ng/mL

- Directly related to the amount of iron in storage
- Increased in chronic illness, malignancy, and chronic transfusions
- Decreased in malnutrition

Gamma-Glutamyl Transferase (GGT)

0–3 wk	0–130 Units/L
3 wk–3 mo	4–120 Units/L
>3 mo (male)	5–65 Units/L
(female)	5–35 Units/L
1–15 yr	0–23 Units/L
Adult (male)	11–50 Units/L
(female)	7–32 Units/L

- Major sources: liver, kidney, prostate, and spleen
- Increased in biliary obstruction, malignant tumor, and alcohol abuse

Glucose

Term	40–110 mg/dL
1 wk–16 yr	60–105 mg/dL
Adult	70–110 mg/dL

- Most common reason for persistent increase is diabetes mellitus
  - Mild diabetic acidosis   300–450 mg/dL
  - Moderate diabetic acidosis   450–600 mg/dL
  - Severe diabetic acidosis   ≥600 mg/dL
  - Decreased with too little food intake and increased exercise
  - Spills into the urine when blood glucose ranges from 160–190 mg/dL

Hemoglobin A$_{1c}$

All ages   5%–7.5%

- Indication of blood sugar control over time

Iron (Serum)

Newborn	100–250 µg/dL
Infant	40–100 µg/dL
Child	50–120 µg/dL
Adolescent (male)	50–160 µg/dL
(female)	40–150 µg/dL
Adult	50–150 µg/dL (male slightly increased)

- Evening levels are lower, so draw in morning
- Should have no iron supplements for 24 hours before test
- Decreased in iron-deficiency anemia

Lead (Pb)

Class

I	≤ 9 µg/dL	Low risk; retest at 2 years of age
IIA	10–14 µg/dL	Borderline: retest every 3–4 months until three results are <15 µg/dL, then test annually
IIB	15–19 µg/dL	Retest every 2 months
III	20–44 µg/dL	Need medical evaluation; test for iron-deficiency anemia; environmental sources need to be identified and eliminated; may need pharmacologic treatment
IV	45–69 µg/dL	Need medical treatment, environmental assessment, and remediation within 48 hours
V	≥ 70 µg/dL	Need medical treatment, environmental assessment, and remediation immediately

(Gunn and Nechyna, 2003.)

Fingerstick lead levels that are elevated need to be reconfirmed by venipuncture.

Magnesium

1.5–2 mEq/L

- Increased in renal failure and in patients receiving intravenous (IV) magnesium sulfate
- Decreased in chronic malnutrition, chronic aminoglycoside use, and chronic hypercalcemia

Phosphorus

Newborn	4.2–9.5 mg/dL
Infant	4.5–6.5 mg/dL

Child   3.5–6 mg/dL
Adult   2.7–4.5 mg/dL

- Increased in renal failure and vitamin D toxicity
- Decreased in malabsorption
- Most frequent and dangerous electrolyte disorder in hyperalimentation

Potassium (K)

<10 days   4.0–6.0 mEq/L
>10 days   3.5–5.0 mEq/L

- Increased in patients with inadequate renal output
- Decreased in patients with loss through the gastrointestinal (GI) tract from vomiting and nasogastric (NG) tube drainage
- Small changes have a great effect on cardiac muscle
- Hemolysis from squeezing finger or heel can falsely elevate results

Prealbumin

Newborn–6 wk   4–36 mg/dL
6 wk–16 yr   13–27 mg/dL
Adult   18–45 mg/dL

- Used to aid in nutritional assessment
- Decreased in malnutrition

Reticulocyte Count (Retic)

Newborn   3%–7%
1 mo   0.1%–1.7%
2–6 mo   0.7%–2.3%
2–18 yr   0.5%–1.0%
Adult (male)   0.8%–2.5%
       (female) 0.8%–4.1%

- Are less mature RBCs
- Measure bone marrow function
- Increases result from increased destruction and the need for more RBCs from hemolysis of ABO incompatibility and sickle cell disease, or from increased loss from acute blood loss
- Will increase after treatment for iron-deficiency anemia is begun
- Decreased in abnormal bone marrow function

Sodium (Na)

135–145 mEq/L

- Changes not commonly seen because its concentration is always corre-lated with fluid balance
- Elevated in hypertonic dehydration with loss of large amounts of water without proportional losses of sodium
- Decreased in water intoxication in which loss of sodium and water is replaced with water only

Triglycerides (Fasting)

Age	Male (mg/dL)	Female (mg/dL)
0–5 yr	30–86	32–99
6–11 yr	31–108	35–114
12–15 yr	36–138	41–138
16–19 yr	40–163	40–128
20–29 yr	44–185	40–128
Over 29 yr	40–160	35–135

- Increased in nephrotic syndrome, hypothyroidism, and diabetes
- Decrease is rarely a problem

Uric Acid (Serum)

0–2 yr	2.4–4.6 mg/dL
2–12 yr	2.4–5.9 mg/dL
12–14 yr	2.4–6.4 mg/dL
Adult (male)	3.5–7.2 mg/dL
(female)	2.4–6.4 mg/dL

- Increased in gout, renal impairment, eclampsia, neoplastic disease, chemotherapy, radiation, and chronic malnutrition
- Decreased in syndrome of inappropriate antidiuretic hormone (SIADH), renal tubular defects, and liver disease

Urinalysis (UA)

Color	Light yellow to dark amber
Clarity	Should be clear
Odor	Fresh specimen should not have ammonia odor
PH	4.3–8, average 6; is affected by diet; most bacteria (except *Escherichia* coli) increase the pH, creating alkaline urine
Specific gravity (sp. gr.)	Infants–2 years 1.001–1.018
	Adults 1.001–1.040 (usually 1.015–1.025)
	If fixed at 1.010 (sp. gr. of plasma), the kidney has lost the ability to concentrate urine

	The higher the number, the more concentrated the urine
Protein	Usually negative; persistent proteinuria is indicative of renal dysfunction
Sugar	Usually negative; if positive, blood glucose is at least 160 mg/dL
Ketone	Negative; if positive, body is burning fat for energy
Nitrites and leukocyte esterase (LE)	Should be negative; if positive, usually has a urinary tract infection (UTI)
Bilirubin	Negative; if positive, is the first indication of liver disease before jaundice
Urobilinogen	Increased in hemolytic disease
Sediment	Crystals—Uric acid, calcium oxalate, and triple phosphates are normal
	Casts—Most are pathologic; a few hyaline casts are normal; WBC casts (>4–5) are associated with infection; RBC casts are associated with damage to the glomerular membrane

Zinc

70–150 μg/dL

- Major sources: liver and organs, muscles, bones, RBCs, and WBCs
- Increased in copper deficiency
- Decreased in iron-deficiency anemia

CONVERSION TABLES FOR COMMONLY USED APPROXIMATE EQUIVALENTS

1 gram (g)	=	1,000 milligrams (mg)
1 g	=	1 cubic centimeter (cc)
1 mg	=	1/65 grains
1 g	=	15 or 16 grains (gr)
60 or 65 mg	=	1 gr
1 mg	=	1,000 micrograms (μg)
1 kilogram (kg)	=	1,000 g
1 kg	=	2.2 pounds
1 milliliter (mL)	=	1 cc
1 mL	=	15 or 16 minims
1 drop (gtt.)	=	1 minim
4 mL	=	1 dram (fluid dram)
5 mL	=	1 teaspoon (tsp)

15 mL	= 1 tablespoon (Tbsp)
30 mL	= 1 ounce (fluid ounce) (oz)
500 mL	= 1 pint (pt)
1,000 mL	= 1 liter (L)
1 L	= 1 quart (qt)
1 inch (in.)	= 2.54 centimeters (cm)
1 cm	= 10 millimeters (mm)

For quick *rough* conversions without using a calculator:

Pounds to kg: Subtract the first number in the pounds (or first 2 numbers if weight is greater than 100) from the total pounds and divide by 2.

> **Example:** Weight = 45 pounds
> 45 − 4 = 41
> 41 ÷ 2 = 20.5 kg (rough conversion) vs.
> 45 ÷ 2.2 = 20.45 (calculator result)
> Weight = 132 pounds
> 132 − 13 = 119
> 119 ÷ 2 = 59.5 kg (rough conversion) vs.
> 132 ÷ 2.2 = 60 (calculator result)

ABBREVIATIONS COMMONLY USED IN PEDIATRIC NURSING

A2	aortic second sound
AAL	anterior axillary line
AAO × 3	awake, alert, and oriented to person, place, and time
ABD	abdominal
ABG	arterial blood gas
AC > BC	air conduction greater than bone conduction
ACE	angiotensin-converting enzyme
ACTH	adrenocorticotropic hormone
ADD/ADHD	attention deficit disorder/attention deficit hyperactivity disorder
ADH	antidiuretic hormone
ADL	activities of daily living
AFB	acid-fast bacillus
AGN	acute glomerulonephritis
AgNO$_3$	silver nitrate
AIDS	acquired immune deficiency syndrome
ALL	acute lymphoblastic leukemia
ALT	alanine aminotransferase (SGPT)
ALTE	apparent life-threatening event

AML	acute myelogenous leukemia
ANA	antinuclear antibody
ANC	absolute neutrophil count
AOM	acute otitis media
AP	anteroposterior
AS	aortic stenosis
ASA	acetylsalicylic acid (aspirin)
ASD	atrial septal defect
ASO	antistreptolysin-O
AST	aspartate aminotransferase (SGOT)
A-V	atrioventricular
AV	arteriovenous
A&W	alive and well
AZT	zidovudine
BAL	dimercaprol
BC	blood culture
BCS	battered child syndrome
BCP	birth control pills
b.i.d.	two times per day
BiPAP	bilevel positive airway pressure
BM	bowel movement
BOE	bilateral otitis externa
BOM	bilateral otitis media
BOMA	bilateral otitis media, acute
BP	blood pressure
BPD	bronchopulmonary dysplasia
bpm	beats per minute
BRATS	bananas, rice, applesauce, toast, saltines
BS	bowel sounds
BSA	body surface area
BSE	breast self-examination
BUN	blood urea nitrogen
Ca	calcium
calcium EDTA	calcium disodium edetate
CAT	computerized axial tomography
CBC	complete blood count
CCB	calcium channel blocker
CDC	Centers for Disease Control and Prevention
CF	cystic fibrosis
CFU	colony-forming unit
CHD	congenital heart disease
	cyanotic heart disease

CHF	congestive heart failure
CHL	conductive hearing loss
CL	central line
cm	centimeter
CMV	cytomegalovirus
CNS	central nervous system
CO	carbon monoxide
CO_2	carbon dioxide
CoA	coarctation of aorta
CP	cerebral palsy
CPAP	continuous positive airway pressure
CPK	creatinine phosphokinase
CPR	cardiopulmonary resuscitation
Cr	creatinine
C&S	culture and sensitivity
CSF	cerebrospinal fluid
C-spine	cervical spine
CT	computed tomography
CTA	clear to auscultation
CVA	costovertebral angle
CVL	central venous line
c/w	compared with
CXR	chest x ray
dc	discharge
D/C	discontinue
DDAVP	desmopressin
DDH	developmental dysplasia of the hip
DEA	Drug Enforcement Agency
DIC	disseminated intravascular coagulation
diff	differential
DKA	diabetic ketoacidosis
dl or dL	deciliter
DM	diabetes mellitus
DNA	deoxyribonucleic acid
DNR	do not resuscitate
DOB	date of birth
DOE	dyspnea on exertion
DTaP	diphtheria-tetanus-acellular pertussis (vaccine)
DTP	diphtheria-tetanus-pertussis (vaccine)
DTR	deep tendon reflex
DVT	deep vein thrombosis
D_5W	5% dextrose in water
$D_{25}W$	25% dextrose in water

Dx	diagnosis
EBV	Epstein-Barr virus
ECD	endocardial cushion defect
ECG/EKG	electrocardiogram
ECHO	echocardiogram
ED	emergency department
EDTA	ethylenediaminetetraacetic acid
EEG	electroencephalogram
ELISA	enzyme-linked immunosorbent assay
EM	erythema multiforme
ENT	ear, nose, and throat
EOM	extraocular movement
EOS	eosinophil
ESR	erythrocyte sedimentation rate
ET	endotracheal
ETT	endotracheal tube
FB	foreign body
FBS	fasting blood sugar
FDA	Food and Drug Administration
Fe	iron
FEV_1	forced expiratory volume in one second
FH_X	family history
FOC	formula of choice
	frontal occipital circumference
FROM	full range of motion
FSH	follicle-stimulating hormone
FTT	failure to thrive
F/U	follow-up
FUO	fever of unknown origin
F_X	fracture
g	gram
GABHS	group A beta hemolytic streptococcus
GC	gonococcal
G-CSF	granulocyte colony-stimulating factor
GE	gastroenteritis
GERD	gastroesophageal reflux disease
GH	growth hormone
GI	gastrointestinal
GnRH	gonadotropin-releasing hormone
gtt.	drops
GTT	glucose tolerance test
	glutamyl transferase
GU	genitourinary

GYN	gynecology
HA	headache
HbA$_{1c}$	glycosylated hemoglobin
HbCV	*Haemophilus influenzae* type b conjugate vaccine
HBIG	hepatitis B immune globulin
HBsAg	hepatitis B surface antigen
HBV	hepatitis B virus
HC	head circumference
hCG	human chorionic gonadotropin
HCO$_3$	bicarbonate
Hct	hematocrit
HDL	high-density lipoprotein
HEENT	head, eyes, ears, nose, and throat
Hg	mercury
Hgb	hemoglobin
HIB	*Haemophilus influenzae* type b (vaccine)
HIV	human immunodeficiency virus
HLA	human lymphocyte antigen
H/O	history of
H$_2$O$_2$	hydrogen peroxide
H&P	history and physical
HPV	human papillomavirus
HR	heart rate
h.s.	at bedtime
HSP	Henoch-Schönlein purpura
HSV	herpes simplex virus
HTN	hypertension
HUS	hemolytic uremic syndrome
H$_X$	history
IBD	inflammatory bowel disease
ICP	intracranial pressure
ICS	intercostal space
I&D	incision and drainage
IDDM	insulin-dependent diabetes mellitus
IDM	infant of a diabetic mother
IgA	immunoglobulin A
IgG	immunoglobulin G
IgM	immunoglobulin M
IGR	intrauterine growth retardation
IID	intermittent infusion device
IM	intramuscular
INH	isoniazid

IO	intraosseous
I&O	intake and output
IPPB	intermittent positive pressure breathing
IPPV	intermittent positive pressure ventilation
IPV	inactivated polio vaccine
ITP	immune thrombocytopenic purpura
IUD	intrauterine device
IUGR	intrauterine growth retardation
IUTD	immunizations up to date
IV	intravenous
IVF	in vitro fertilization
IVIG	intravenous immune globulin
IVP	intravenous pyelogram
JDM	juvenile diabetes mellitus
JRA	juvenile rheumatoid arthritis
K	potassium
Kcal	kilocalorie
KCl	potassium chloride
KD	Kawasaki disease
kg	kilogram
KOH	potassium hydroxide
KUB	kidney, ureter, and bladder
KVO	keep vein open
LDL	low-density lipoprotein
LET	lidocaine, epinephrine, tetracaine
LFTs	liver function tests
LGA	large for gestational age
LH	luteinizing hormone
LIP	lymphoid interstitial pneumonitis
LLE	left lower extremity
LLL	left lower lobe
LLQ	left lower quadrant
LP	lumbar puncture
LTB	laryngotracheobronchitis
LUL	left upper lobe
LUQ	left upper quadrant
max	maximum
MCHC	mean corpuscular hemoglobin concentration
MCL	midclavicular line
MCV	mean corpuscular volume
MDI	metered-dose inhaler
mEq	milliequivalent

mg	milligram
min	minute
ml or mL	milliliter
mm	millimeter
MMR	measles-mumps-rubella (vaccine)
MR	mental retardation
MRI	magnetic resonance imaging
MRSA	methicillin-resistant *Staphylococcus aureus*
MRSE	methicillin-resistant *Staphylococcus epidermidis*
MSBP	Munchausen syndrome by proxy
MTX	methotrexate
Na	sodium
NAD	no acute distress
$NaHCO_3$	sodium bicarbonate
NEC	necrotizing enterocolitis
NF	neurofibromatosis
NFTSD	normal full-term spontaneous delivery
NG	nasogastric
NH_3	ammonia
NIDDM	non-insulin-dependent diabetes mellitus
NKA	no known allergies
NKDA	no known drug allergies
NP	nasopharyngeal
NPO	nothing by mouth
NSAID	nonsteroidal anti-inflammatory drug
NSR	normal sinus rhythm
O_2	oxygen
OCD	obsessive-compulsive disorder
OD	right eye
OM	otitis media
OPV	oral polio vaccine
OS	left eye
OTC	over the counter
OU	each eye
oz	ounce
P	phosphorus
PARA	number of pregnancies
Pb	lead
PBS	phenobarbital sodium
PCA	patient-controlled analgesia
PCN	penicillin
PCOS	polycystic ovarian syndrome

pCO$_2$	partial pressure of carbon dioxide
PCP	*Pneumocystis carinii* pneumonia
PDA	patent ductus arteriosus
PE	physical examination
PEF	peak expiratory flow
PEFR	peak expiratory flow rate
PERRLA	pupils equal, round, and reactive to light and accommodation
PET	positron emission tomography
PFM	peak flow meter
PGG	pH, glucose, guaiac
PID	pelvic inflammatory disease
PKU	phenylketonuria
PMI	point of maximal impulse
PNET	primitive neuroectodermal tumor
PO	by mouth
Po$_2$	partial pressure of oxygen
PO$_4$	phosphate
PPD	purified protein derivative (used in tuberculosis skin test)
PPS	post-pericardial syndrome
p.r.n.	as needed
pt	patient
PT	prothrombin time
PTA	prior to admission
PTSD	post-traumatic stress disorder
PTT	partial thromboplastin time
PUD	peptic ulcer disease
PVC	premature ventricular contraction
PVR	postvoiding residual
q	every
q.i.d.	four times per day
QOL	quality of life
RA	rheumatoid arthritis
RAD	reactive airway disease
RBC	red blood cell
RDS	respiratory distress syndrome
REM	rapid eye movement
RF	rheumatic fever
RLE	right lower extremity
RLL	right lower lobe
RLQ	right lower quadrant

RML	right middle lobe
RMSF	Rocky Mountain spotted fever
R/O	rule out
ROM	range of motion
	right otitis media
ROS	rule out sepsis
RR	respiratory rate
RSV	respiratory syncytial virus
RUQ	right upper quadrant
RVH	right ventricular hypertrophy
R_X	prescription
S1	first heart sound
S2	second heart sound
S3	third heart sound
S4	fourth heart sound
SaO_2	oxygen saturation
SB	spina bifida
	sternal border
SBE	subacute bacterial endocarditis
SCC	sickle cell crisis
SCD	sickle cell disease
SCFE	slipped capital femoral epiphysis
SGA	small for gestational age
SGOT	serum glutamic oxaloacetic transaminase (AST)
SGPT	serum glutamic pyruvic transaminase (ALT)
SIADH	syndrome of inappropriate antidiuretic hormone
SIDS	sudden infant death syndrome
sig.	directions
SLE	systemic lupus erythematosus
SO	significant other
SOB	shortness of breath
SOM	serous otitis media
S/P	status post
sp. gr.	specific gravity
SSD	sickle cell disease
STD	sexually transmitted disease
S_X	symptoms
T	temperature
T_3	triiodothyronine
T_4	tetraiodothyronine
T&A	tonsillectomy and adenoidectomy
TAC	tetracaine, adrenaline (epinephrine), and cocaine

TB	tuberculosis
TEF	tracheoesophageal fistula
TGA	transposition of the great arteries
TGV	transposition of the great vessels
t.i.d.	three times per day
TM	tympanic membrane
TOF	tetralogy of Fallot
TORCH	toxoplasmosis, other infections, rubella, cytomegalovirus, and herpes simplex
TPA	total parenteral alimentation
TPN	total parenteral nutrition
TRH	thyroid-releasing hormone
TSH	thyroid-stimulating hormone
tsp	teaspoon
T_X	treatment
UA	urinalysis
URI	upper respiratory infection
US	ultrasound
USOH	usual state of health
UTD	up to date
UTI	urinary tract infection
VCUG	voiding cystourethrogram
VP	ventriculoperitoneal
vs	versus
VS	vital signs
VSD	ventricular septal defect
VSS	vital signs stable
WBC	white blood cell
WHO	World Health Organization
w/u	work-up

In response to patient safety concerns, the Joint Commission on Accreditation of Healthcare Organizations (JCAHO) has established a "do not use" list of abbreviations. The following abbreviations are included on the "do not use" list: U (unit), IU (International Unit), Q.D. (daily), Q.O.D. (every other day), MS (morphine sulfate or magnesium sulfate), MSO_4 (morphine sulfate), and $MgSO_4$ (magnesium sulfate).

CHAPTER 4

DRUG ADMINISTRATION

COMMON PEDIATRIC DRUGS

Efforts have been made to ensure that drug dosage information herein is accurate and reflects acceptable standards at the time of publication. However, changes in practice continually occur. Therefore, readers are advised to check product information included with each drug to be sure that changes have not been made.

Estimates of Weight Per Age

It is essential to obtain an accurate weight (in kilograms) of the child upon admission and then periodically during prolonged admissions. Pediatric dosages are calculated based upon the child's weight (in kilograms). If the child's weight is not available, it is possible to estimate the weight based upon age.

WEIGHT PER AGE ESTIMATES	
Age	Weight in kg
6 mo	7
1 yr	10
2–3 yr	12–14
3–4 yr	14–16
5–6 yr	18–20
7–8 yr	22–24
9–10 yr	28–34
11–12 yr	40–45
13–14 yr	47–50

acetaminophen (Tylenol, Tempra, and others)

Indications

(analgesic; antipyretic)

Mild to moderate pain, fever.

Administration

10–15 mg/kg/dose q4–6h; 5 doses in 24 hr (max. dose: 4 g/24 hr, 5 doses/24 hr)

Dosing by age: PO or PR

0–3 mo:	40 mg/dose
4–11 mo:	80 mg/dose
12–24 mo:	120 mg/dose
2–3 yr:	160 mg/dose
4–5 yr:	240 mg/dose
6–8 yr:	320 mg/dose
9–10 yr:	400 mg/dose
11–12 yr:	480 mg/dose
Adult:	325–650 mg/dose

Nursing Implications

Dose standardization common. Contraindicated in known glucose-6-phosphate dehydrogenase (G6PD) deficiency. Rectal absorption variable. Use cautiously in severe hepatic disease. Administer with food to decrease gastrointestinal (GI) upset. Assess and document effect 30–60 min after administration. Can cause rash, blood dyscrasias.

acetylcysteine (Mucomyst, Mucosil)

Indications

(mucolytic; antidote)

Used for treatment of abnormally viscid mucous secretions as a result of acute and chronic respiratory disease. Other uses include treatment of pulmonary complications of cystic fibrosis, tracheostomy care, and acetaminophen (Tylenol) overdose.

Administration

Reduction of pulmonary secretion viscosity:

Children:	Nebulize 3–5 mL of 20% solution t.i.d. or q.i.d.
	Nebulize 6–10 mL of 10% solution t.i.d. or q.i.d.
Infants:	Nebulize 1–2 mL of 20% solution t.i.d. or q.i.d.
	Nebulize 2–4 mL of 10% solution t.i.d. or q.i.d.
Intratracheal instillation:	1–2 mL of 10%–20% solution instilled into tracheostomy q1–4 hr
Acetaminophen poisoning:	5% solution of 140 mg/kg PO followed by 70 mg/kg for 17 doses q4h until acetaminophen levels are nontoxic

Nursing Implications

Slight odor from solution may be noticed during initial administration but quickly disappears. Dilute with juice or soda when giving PO.

acyclovir (Zovirax)

Indications

(antiviral agent)

Used in treatment of herpes simplex virus (HSV) and varicella-zoster virus in healthy, nonpregnant ≥13 yr olds. Also used in children ≥12 mo with immune or chronic disorders.

Administration

HSV:
    Initial infection:
        IV: 15 mg/kg/24 hr ÷ q8h × 5–7 days
        PO: 1,200 mg/24 hr ÷ q8h × 7–10 days
    Recurrence:
        PO: 1,200 mg/24 hr ÷ q8h *or* 1,600 mg/24 hr ÷ q12h
                        × 5 days
    Neonatal HSV
        and HSV
        encephalitis:
        All ages: 30 mg/kg/24 hr ÷ q8h IV × 14–21 days
    Term infants can have higher doses of 45–60 mg/kg/24 hr ÷ q8h IV
Zoster:
    IV: 30 mg/kg/24 hr ÷ q8h × 7–10 days
    PO: 4,000 mg/24 hr ÷ 5x/24 hr × 5–7 days for
                        patients ≥12 yr
Varicella:
    IV: 30 mg/kg/24 hr ÷ q8h × 7–10 days
    PO: 80 mg/kg/24 hr ÷ q.i.d. × 5 days (start within 24 hr
                        of rash onset) (max. dose: 3,200 mg/24 hr)
                        (max. dose of oral acyclovir in children is
                        80 mg/kg/24 hr)
IV dilution:
    Max.
        concentration: 7–10 mg/mL
    Usual
        concentration: 10 mg/mL over 60 min
Compatibility: 5% dextrose in water (D_5W), normal saline (NS), lactated ringers (LR)

Nursing Implications

Adequate hydration and slow IV administration essential to prevent crystal formation in renal tubules. Dose reduction required in renal impairment. Side effects include headache (HA), lethargy, skin rash, nausea, vomiting, and bone marrow suppression.

albuterol (Proventil, Ventolin)

Indications

(β_2-adrenergic agent)

Bronchodilator used in asthma or reactive airway disease (RAD) for prevention and relief of bronchospasm.

Administration

PO:

<6 yr:	0.3 mg/kg/24 hr ÷ q8h (max. dose: 12 mg/24 hr)
6–11 yr:	6 mg/24 hr ÷ t.i.d. (max. dose: 24 mg/24 hr)
≥12 yr/adult:	2–4 mg dose t.i.d.–q.i.d. (max. dose: 32 mg/24 hr)

Inhalations:

Aerosol (metered-dose inhaler [MDI]):	1–2 puffs (90–180 μg) q4–6h p.r.n.

Nebulized:

<1 yr:	0.05–0.15 mg/kg/dose q4–6h
1–5 yr:	1.25–2.5 mg/dose q4–6h
5–12 yr:	2.5 mg/dose q6h
>12 yr:	2.5–5 mg/dose q6h

Higher doses can be used in acute exacerbations.

Nursing Implications

Administer PO with meals to decrease gastric irritation. Use spacer with MDI to enhance efficacy. Side effects include tachycardia, palpitations, tremor, insomnia, nervousness, nausea, and HA. Side effects more pronounced with PO doses, less with nebulizer, and least with MDI.

allopurinol (Zyloprim and others)

Indications

(uric acid lowering agent; xanthine oxidase inhibitor)

Used to prevent attacks of gouty arthritis and nephropathy. Also used to treat secondary hyperuricemia and for prevention of recurrent calcium oxalate calculi.

Administration

Child: 10 mg/kg/24 hr ÷ b.i.d.–q.i.d. PO (max. dose: 800 mg/24 hr)
Adult: 200–300 mg/24 hr ÷ b.i.d.–t.i.d. PO

Nursing Implications

Side effects include rash, neuritis, hepatotoxicity, GI disturbances, bone marrow suppression, and drowsiness.

amikacin (Amikin)

Indications

(antibiotic; aminoglycoside)

Used in treatment of serious gram-negative bacillary infections and staphylococcal infections when penicillin and other less toxic drugs are contraindicated.

Administration

Infant or child:	15–22.5 mg/kg/24 hr ÷ q8h IV/IM
Adult:	15 mg/kg/24 hr ÷ q8–12h IV/IM (max. dose: 1.5 g/24 hr, then monitor levels)
IV dilution:	5 mg/mL over 30–60 min; 50 mg/mL central venous line (CVL)
Compatibility:	D₅W, NS, LR

Nursing Implications

Therapeutic levels must be monitored. Peak: 20–30 mg/L; trough: 5–10 mg/L. Dose adjusted in renal insufficiency. Patient needs to be well hydrated. May cause ototoxicity, nephrotoxicity, neuromuscular blockade, and rash.

amiodarone hydrochloride (Cordarone)

Indications

(antiarrhythmic agent, class III)

Used to manage resistant, life-threatening ventricular arrhythmias unresponsive to conventional treatment with less toxic agents.

Administration

Child PO:

<1 yr:	600–800 mg/1.73m²/24 hr ÷ q12–24h, then decrease to 200–400 mg/1.73m²/24 hr
≥1 yr:	10–15 mg/kg/24 hr ÷ q12–24h × 4–14 days or until adequate control is achieved, then decrease to 5 mg/kg/24 hr ÷ q12–24h

Child IV: (limited data available) 5 mg/kg over 30 min followed by a continuous infusion starting at 5μg/kg/min; may be increased to a max. dose of 10μg/kg/min *or* 20 mg/kg/24 hr

IV dilution: 2 mg/mL *or* 6 mg/mL CVL

Compatibility: D_5W

Nursing Implications

Proposed therapeutic levels with chronic oral use is 1–2.5 mg/L. Side effects include asymptomatic corneal microdeposits, altered liver enzymes, paresthesias, ataxia, tremor, and hyperthyroidism or hypothyroidism.

amitriptyline (Elavil, Emitrip, Endep, Enovil)

Indications

(tricyclic antidepressant; antimigraine agent)

Used to treat various forms of depression, as an analgesic for certain chronic and neuropathic pain, and as a migraine prophylaxis. Unlabeled use—treatment of bulimia.

Administration

Chronic pain
  management:
  Child: Initially 0.1 mg/kg q.h.s. PO; may increase over 2–3 wk to 0.5–2 mg/kg q.h.s. PO

Antidepressant:
  Child: 1 mg/kg/24 hr ÷ t.i.d. PO × 3 days, then increase to 1.5 mg/kg/24 hr (max. dose: 5 mg/kg/24 hr)

  Adolescent: 10 mg t.i.d. with 20 mg q.h.s. PO (max. dose: 200 mg/24 hr)

  Adult: 30–100 mg/24 hr q.h.s.–b.i.d. PO (max. dose: 300 mg/24 hr)

    20–30 mg q.i.d. IM (convert to PO as soon as possible)

Nursing Implications

Monitor electrocardiogram (ECG), blood pressure (BP), and heart rate (HR) for doses >3 mg/kg/24 hr. Maximum antidepressant effect takes 2 wk. Therapeutic level is 120–250 ng/mL and is checked 8 hr after PO dose and after 4–5 days of continuous dosing. Side effects include sedation, urinary retention, constipation, dry mouth, dizziness, drowsiness, and arrhythmia. Do not give IV. May administer with food to decrease GI upset.

amoxicillin (Amoxil, Trimox, Wymox, Polymox)

Indications

(antibiotic; aminopenicillin)

Used in treatment of a variety of infections including, most commonly, otitis media (OM), as a first-line drug. Also used in sinusitis, respiratory and genitourinary (GU) tract infections, and for subacute bacterial endocarditis (SBE) prophylaxis. Unlabeled use—treatment of Lyme disease.

Administration

Child: 20 -50 mg/kg/24 hr ÷ q8h PO of 125- or 250-mg/5 cc strength *or* 25–45 mg/kg/24 hr ÷ b.i.d. PO of 200- or 400-mg/5 cc strength

Higher doses of 75–90 mg/kg/24 hr ÷ t.i.d. have been recommended for treatment of resistant *Streptococcus pneumoniae* in OM.

Adult: 250–500 mg/dose q8h PO (max. dose: 2–3 g/24 hr)

Endocarditis

prophylaxis: 50 mg/kg 1 hr before procedure (not to exceed adult dose)

Nursing Implications

Most common side effects are rashes and diarrhea. Food does not interfere with absorption.

amoxicillin/clavulanate (Augmentin)

Indications

(antibiotic; aminopenicillin with β-lactamase inhibitor)

Same as amoxicillin but extends its activity to include β-lactamase-producing strains of *Haemophilus influenzae* and *Branhamella (Neisseria) catarrhalis.*

Administration

Child <3 mo: 30 mg/kg/24 hr ÷ b.i.d. PO using 125-mg/5 cc strength

Child ≥3 mo, <40 kg: 20–40 mg/kg/24 hr ÷ t.i.d. PO of 125- or 250-mg/ 5 cc strength *or*
25–45 mg/kg/24 hr ÷ b.i.d. PO of 200- or 400-mg/ 5 cc strength

Adult: 250–500 mg/dose q8h PO *or* 875 mg q12h PO (max. dose: 2g/24 hr)

Nursing Implications

Incidence of diarrhea higher than with amoxicillin, but lower with b.i.d. dosing strength and schedule. Give with meals to help decrease GI side effects.

amphotericin B (Fungizone, Amphocin)

Indications

(antifungal; antiprotozoal)

Used in treatment of severe systemic infections and meningitis caused by susceptible fungi.

Administer

Topical: Apply b.i.d.–t.i.d.
PO: 100 mg q.i.d. for oral candidiasis
IV:

    Test dose: 0.1 mg/kg/dose up to max. of 1 mg (followed by remaining initial dose)

    Initial dose: 0.25–0.5 mg/kg/24 hr

    Increment: Increase as tolerated by 0.25–0.5 mg/kg/24 hr daily or every other day

    Maintenance: 0.25–1 mg/kg/24 hr *or* 1.5 mg/kg/dose every other day (max. dose: 1.5 mg/kg/24 hr)

IV dilution: Mix to concentration of 0.1 mg/mL (peripheral) *or* 0.2 mg/mL (CVL) over 2–6 hr

Compatibility: D_5W

Nursing Implications

Common infusion-related reactions are fever, chills, HA, hypotension, nausea, and vomiting. May need to premedicate with acetaminophen and diphenhydramine HCI (Benadryl) 30 min before and 4 hr after infusion.

ampicillin (Omnipen, Polycillin, Principen, Totacillin-N)

Indications

(antibiotic; aminopenicillin)

Used for treatment of OM, sinusitis, respiratory tract infections, GU infections, meningitis, septicemia, and suspected group B streptococcal infections as well as for endocarditis prophylaxis.

Administration

Neonate:

    <7days, <2 kg: 50–100 mg/kg/24 hr ÷ q12h IV/IM

    <7 days, ≥2 kg: 75–150 mg/kg/24 hr ÷ q8h IV/IM

    ≥7 days, <1.2 kg: 50–100 mg/kg/24 hr ÷ q12h IV/IM

    ≥7 days, 1.2–2 kg: 75–150 mg/kg/24 hr ÷ q8h IV/IM

    ≥7 days, > 2 kg: 100–200 mg/kg/24 hr ÷ q6h IV/IM

Child:
Mild to moderate infections:	100–200 mg/kg/24 hr ÷ q6h IV/IM
	50–100 mg/kg/24 hr ÷ q6h PO (max. PO dose: 2–3g/24 hr)
Severe infections:	200–400 mg/kg/24 hr ÷ q4–6h IV/IM (max. IV/IM dose: 12g/24 hr)
Adult:	500–3,000 mg q4–6h IV/IM
	250–500 mg q6h PO
IV dilution:	
Direct IV:	Up to 500 mg only, over 3–5 min
	>500 mg, over 10–15 min
	(max. concentration 100 mg/mL; not to exceed 100 mg/min)
Intermittent IV:	30 mg/mL over 15–30 min
Compatibility:	D₅W, NS preferred, LR, sterile water (SW)

Nursing Implications

Higher doses used to treat central nervous system (CNS) disease. Hypersensitivity rash commonly seen at 5–10 days. Administer PO dose with water on an empty stomach 1–2 hr before meals. Reconstituted ampicillin sodium effective for 1 hr after reconstitution. IV administration at >100 mg/min may cause seizures. Can also cause interstitial nephritis, diarrhea, and pseudomembranous enterocolitis.

ampicillin/sulbactam (Unasyn)
Indications

(antibiotic; aminopenicillin with β-lactamase inhibitor)
    Used to treat susceptible bacterial infections involved with skin, abdominal, and gynecologic infections. Effective against β-lactamase-producing organisms.

Administration

(dosage based on ampicillin component)
Child:
Mild to moderate infections:	100–200 mg/kg/24 hr ÷ q6h IV/IM
Severe infections:	200–400 mg/kg/24 hr ÷ q4–6h IV/IM
Adult:	1–2 g q6–8h IV/IM (max. dose: 8g ampicillin/24 hr)
IV dilution:	Max. concentration 45 mg of Unasyn/mL over 10–15 min
Compatibility:	D₅W, NS

Nursing Implications

Dose adjusted in renal failure. Similar cerebrospinal fluid (CSF) distribution and side effects as ampicillin.

aspirin, acetylsalicylic acid, ASA (Ecotrin, Bufferin, Bayer, and others)

Indications

(nonsteroidal anti-inflammatory drug [NSAID]; antiplatelet agent; analgesic) Mild pain and fever. Also useful as an antipyretic and in Kawasaki disease.

Administration

Analgesic or antipyretic: 10–15 mg/kg/dose q4h PO/PR up to a total of
                            60–80 mg/kg/24 hr (max. dose: 4g/24 hr)
Anti-inflammatory: 60–100 mg/kg/24 hr ÷ q6–8h PO
Kawasaki disease: 80–100 mg/kg/24 hr ÷ q.i.d. PO during febrile
                            phase, then decrease to 3–5 mg/kg/24 hr q AM PO

Nursing Implications

Do not use in children <16 yr old with chickenpox or flu-like symptoms because of risk for Reye's syndrome. Use with caution in GI disease. May cause GI upset, tinnitus, allergic reactions, liver toxicity, and platelet aggregation. Give with water, food, or milk to decrease GI upset. Therapeutic levels vary according to purpose of administration; consult laboratory.

atenolol (Tenolin, Tenormin)

Indications

(beta$_1$-adrenergic blocker; antihypertensive; antianginal; antiarrhythmic)
     Used for treatment of hypertension. May be used as single agent or combined with other antihypertensives.

Administration

PO:
   Child: Initially 0.8–1 mg/kg/day in single dose. Dosage
                            may be increased to 1.5 mg/kg/day (max. daily
                            dosage of 2 mg/kg/day)

Nursing Implications

Monitor for hypotension, complaints of dizziness, and nausea. Medication should not be abruptly discontinued. Therapeutic antihypertensive effects usually are noted within 1–2 weeks.

atomoxetine (Strattera)

Indications

(nonstimulant; norepinephrine reuptake inhibitor)

Used to treat patients 6 years and older with attention deficit hyperactivity disorder.

Administration

Children > 70 kg: 40 mg PO once daily (may increase after 3 days to
                  80 mg PO daily)
                  Maximum daily dose: 100 mg PO
Children < 70 kg: Initially, 0.5 mg/kg/day PO (may increase to
                  1.2 mg/kg/day after 3 days)
                  Maximum daily dose: 1.4 mg/kg/day PO

Nursing Implications

GI side effects such as nausea, vomiting, and dyspepsia are common. Reduced appetite and weight loss may occur.

atropine sulfate (Atropair)

Indications

(anticholinergic; parasympatholytic)

Used to prevent or reduce salivation and respiratory tract secretions in anesthesia. Also used to treat symptomatic bradycardia and to restore normal heart contraction during cardiac arrest. Increases HR and cardiac output by blocking vagal stimulation in the heart.

Administration

Preoperative: 0.02 mg/kg SQ/IM/IV to a maximum dose of
                about 1 mg given 30–60 minutes prior to induction of
                anesthesia
Bradycardia: 0.02 mg/kg IV, IO, ET with a minimum dose of 0.1 mg
                and maximum dose of 0.5 mg in children, 1 mg in
                adolescents, and 2 mg in adults (repeat q5min to
                max total dose of 1 mg in children and 2 mg in
                adolescents)
Compatibility: Incompatible with sodium bicarbonate and
                epinephrine

Nursing Implications

Effect on HR occurs in 2–4 minutes. Continuous monitoring of vital signs is necessary.

azathioprine (Imuran)

Indications

(immunosuppressant)
 Used to prevent rejection in kidney transplantation.

Administration

Kidney transplantation:	3–5 mg/kg/day IV as single dose on day of transplant
	3–5 mg/kg/day PO before or at the time of surgery
	1–3 mg/kg/day PO as maintenance dose
IV dilution:	Reconstitute 100 mg vial with 10 mL of sterile water
	May further dilute in 50 mL compatible fluid. Infuse for 30–60 minutes
Compatibility:	D$_5$W, 0.9% NS

Nursing Implications

Metabolism of azathioprine is decreased by allopurinol so lower dosages are needed. Frequent side effects are nausea, vomiting, and anorexia (especially during early phase of treatment). CBC, platelet count, and LFTs should be performed q week during first month of therapy, twice monthly during second and third months of treatment, and then monthly thereafter.

azithromycin (Zithromax)

Indications

(antibiotic; macrolide)
 Used to treat mild to moderate upper and lower respiratory infections, skin infections, acute OM, and sexually transmitted diseases (STDs).

Administration

Child:

OM or community-acquired pneumonia (≥6 mo):	10 mg/kg on day 1 daily PO (max. dose: 500 mg), then 5 mg/kg on days 2–5 daily PO (max. dose: 250 mg)
Pharyngitis or tonsillitis (≥2 yr):	12 mg/kg/24 hr daily PO (max. dose: 500 mg/24 hr)

Adolescent or adult:

Respiratory tract, skin, and soft-tissue infection:	500 mg on day 1 daily PO, then 250 mg on days 2–5 daily PO
Acute pelvic inflammatory disease (PID):	500 mg daily IV × 1–2 days, then 250 mg daily PO to complete 7- to 10-day therapy

IV dilution: 1 mg/mL over 3 hr *or* 2 mg/mL over
                                          1 hr. Do not infuse over a
                                          period <60 min.
Compatibility: NaCl, D$_5$W

Nursing Implications

Can cause increase in liver enzymes, cholestatic jaundice, and GI discomfort. Capsules and oral suspension should be administered on an empty stomach, 1 hr before or 2 hr after a meal. Tablets and oral powder (sachet) can be given with food.

beclomethasone dipropionate (Beclovent, Beconase, Beconase AQ, Vanceril, Vancenase, Vancenase AQ)

Indications

(corticosteroid)

Used as inhalation for long-term control of persistent bronchial asthma and intranasally for management of seasonal or perennial rhinitis and nasal polyposis.

Administration

Oral inhalation
  (42 μg/inhalation
  [puff]):
  6–12 yr: 1–2 puffs t.i.d.–q.i.d. *or* 2–4 puffs b.i.d. max. dose:
                                10 puffs/24 hr
  >12 yr: 2 puffs t.i.d.–q.i.d. (max. dose: 12 puffs/24 hr)
Oral inhalation,
  double strength
  (84 μg/puff):
  6–12 yr: 2 puffs b.i.d. (max. dose: 5 puffs/24 hr)
  >12 yr: 2 puffs b.i.d. (max. dose: 10 puffs/24 hr)
Nasal inhalation:
  6–12 yr: 1 spray each nostril t.i.d.
  >12 yr: 1 spray each nostril b.i.d.–q.i.d. *or* 2 sprays each
                                nostril b.i.d.
Aqueous nasal spray:
  >6 yr–adult: 1–2 sprays each nostril b.i.d.

Nursing Implications

Not recommended for use in children <6 yr. *Avoid* using higher-than-recommended doses because they can cause hypothalamic, pituitary, or adrenal suppression. Onset for oral inhalation is 1–4 wk; for nasal inhalation it is a few days to 2 wk. If child objects to the taste, have him or her drink a glass of orange juice before inhaling. Shake nasal and oral inhalation containers well before using. Have child rinse mouth after oral inhalation to prevent thrush. Spacers recommended for oral inhalations to increase amount of medicine getting to lungs. Side effects include HA, sore throat, thrush, cough, sneezing, hoarseness, irritation and burning of the nasal mucosa, nasal ulceration, epistaxis, rhinorrhea, and nasal congestion.

bethanechol chloride (Urecholine)

Implications

(cholinergic agent)

Used in treatment of nonobstructive urinary retention and abdominal distension. Also effective in treatment of gastroesophageal (GE) reflux.

Administration

Child:

Abdominal distension	0.6 mg/kg/24 hr ÷ q6–8h PO
or urinary retention:	0.12–0.2 mg/kg/24 hr ÷ q6–8h SC
GE reflux:	0.1–0.2 mg/kg/dose ÷ q.i.d. (30 min a.c. and h.s.) PO (max. dose: 4 doses in 24 hr)
Adult:	10–50 mg q6–12h PO
	2.5–5 mg t.i.d.–q.i.d. SC, up to 7.5–10 mg q4h SC for neurogenic bladder

Nursing Implications

Contraindicated in asthma, mechanical GI or GU obstruction, peptic ulcer disease, cardiac disease, hyperthyroidism, and seizure disorder. Can cause hypotension; nausea; abdominal cramps; and increased salivation, flushing, and bronchospasm. Administer on empty stomach to reduce nausea and vomiting. Do not give IM or IV.

bisacodyl (Dulcolax)

Indications

(laxative; stimulant)

Used to evacuate colon. Indicated in treatment of constipation associated with bed rest or spinal cord injury. Also used as preparation for surgery or X ray studies.

Administration

PO:

Child:	0.3 mg/kg/24 hr *or* 5–10 mg 6 hr before desired effect
Adult (>12 yr):	5–15 mg daily

PR:

<2 yr:	5 mg
2–11 yr:	5–10 mg
>11 yr:	10 mg

Nursing Implications

Tablets should not be crushed or chewed. Do not give within 1 hr of milk or antacids. Can cause nausea and abdominal cramping. Oral dose effective in 6–10 hr. Rectal effective within 15–60 min.

budesonide (Rhinocort, Pulmicort)
Indications

(glucocorticosteroid; anti-inflammatory; antiallergy)

Used to treat seasonal allergic rhinitis and as maintenance treatment of asthma.

Administration

Intranasal:	2 sprays each nostril b.i.d. (max. dose 8 sprays/day)
Nebulization:	0.25–1 mg/day
Inhalation:	200–400 mcg twice daily

Nursing Implications

Rinse mouth after inhalation use. Side effects include mild nasopharyngeal irritation, burning, stinging, dryness, cough. Improvement of symptoms may be noted in 24 hrs but full effect may take up to 3–7 days.

bumetanide (Bumex)
Indications

(loop diuretic)

Used to treat edema associated with congestive heart failure, chronic renal failure (including nephritic syndrome), and acute pulmonary edema.

Administration

Neonates:	0.01–0.05 mg/kg/dose PO or IV q24–48h
Infants or children:	0.015–0.1 mg/kg/dose PO or IV q6–24h to max. dose of 10 mg/day
IV dilution:	May be given undiluted; adminster IV push >1–2 minutes
Compatibility:	D$_5$W, LR, 0.9% NaCl

Nursing Implications

Give PO dose with food to minimize GI upset. Expected side effect is increase in urine frequency and volume. Other frequent side effects are orthostatic hypotension and dizziness.

calcitriol (Rocaltrol, Calcijex)

Indications

(active form of vitamin D, fat soluble)

Most potent form of vitamin D available. Used most often in management of hypocalcemia in chronic renal failure. Promotes absorption of calcium from GI tract.

Administration

Renal failure:

Child:	Range 0.01–0.05 μg/kg/24 hr PO; is titrated in 0.005- to 0.01-μg/kg/24 hr increments q4–8wk based on clinical response
	0.01–0.05 μg/kg/dose IV 3x/wk
Adult:	Initial dose 0.25 μg/dose PO with increment increase at 0.25 μg/dose PO q4–8wk
	Usual dose 0.5–1 μg/24 hr
	0.5 μg/24 hr IV given 3x/wk
	Usual dose 0.5–3 μg/24 hr IV given 3x/wk
IV dilution:	May be given undiluted as a bolus dose IV at the end of hemodialysis

Nursing Implications

Avoid using with antacids containing magnesium. Contraindicated in patients with hypercalcemia. Serum calcium and phosphorous levels must be monitored. Eating foods high in calcium can lead to hypercalcemia. Can cause weakness, HA, vomiting, constipation, and hypotonia. IV dosing used for patients undergoing hemodialysis.

captopril (Capoten)

Indications

(angiotensin-converting enzyme inhibitor; antihypertensive)

Used in management of hypertension. Also used in combination with other drugs for treatment of congestive heart failure (CHF).

Administration

Neonate:	0.1–0.4 mg/kg/24 hr q6–8h PO

Infant: Initial dose 0.15–0.3 mg/kg/dose PO titrated upward
        for desired effect (max. dose: 6 mg/kg/24 hr ÷
        daily–q.i.d. PO)

Child: Initial dose 0.3–0.5 mg/kg/dose ÷ q8h PO titrated
        upward as needed (max. dose: 6 mg/kg/24 hr ÷
        b.i.d.–q.i.d. PO)

Adolescent or adult: Initial dose 12.5–25 mg/dose b.i.d.–q.i.d. PO increased
        weekly by 25 mg/dose (max. dose: 450 mg/24 hr)

Nursing Implications

Administer on empty stomach 1 hr before or 2 hr after meals. Reaches peak
1–2 hr after administration. Check baseline BP before administration. Use of
NSAIDs may result in reduced antihypertensive response to captopril. May
cause rash, proteinuria, neutropenia, cough, angioedema, hyperkalemia, hypotension, and decreased taste perception with long-term use.

carbamazepine (Tegretol, Carbatrol)

Indications

(anticonvulsant)

Used to prevent tonic-clonic, mixed, and complex partial seizures. Also
used to relieve pain in trigeminal neuralgia or diabetic neuropathy and for
treatment of bipolar disorders.

Administration

Child:

 <6 yr: Initial dose 10–20 mg/kg/24 hr ÷ b.i.d.–t.i.d. PO (q.i.d. for
     suspension)
     Increase at increments q5–7 days up to 35 mg/kg/24 hr PO

 6–12 yr: Initial dose 10 mg/kg/24 hr ÷ b.i.d. up to max. dose of
     100 mg/dose b.i.d. PO
     Increase 100 mg/24 hr at 1-wk intervals ÷ t.i.d.–q.i.d. until
     desired response
     Maintenance dose: 20–30 mg/kg/24 hr ÷ b.i.d.–q.i.d. PO
     Usual maintenance dose: 400–800 mg/24 hr (max. dose:
     1,000 mg/24 hr)

 >12 yr: Initial dose 200 mg b.i.d. PO
     Increase 200 mg/24 hr at 1-wk intervals ÷ b.i.d.–q.i.d. until
     desired response
     Maintenance dose: 800–1,200 mg/24 hr ÷ b.i.d.–q.i.d. PO
     (max. dose: 12–15 yr: 1,000 mg/24 hr; adult: 1.6–2.4 g/
     24 hr)

Nursing Implications

Contraindicated in patients taking monoamine oxidase (MAO) inhibitors. Therapeutic blood levels 4–12 mg/L. Monitoring of serum levels mandatory when patients are switched from any product to another. Erythromycin, isoniazid (INH), cimetidine, and verapamil increase carbamazepine levels. May cause decrease in activity of warfarin, doxycycline, oral contraceptives, cyclosporin, theophylline, phenytoin, benzodiazepines, ethosuximide, and valproic acid. Doses may be administered with food to decrease GI upset. Do not simultaneously administer oral suspension with other liquid medicines or diluents. Side effects include sedation, dizziness, diplopia, aplastic anemia, neutropenia, urinary retention, syndrome of inappropriate antidiuretic hormone (SIADH), and Stevens-Johnson syndrome. Check complete blood cell count (CBC) and liver function tests (LFTs) before course and monitor for hematologic and hepatic toxicity.

carbenicillin (Geocillin, Geopen, Pyopen)

Indications

(antibiotic; extended-spectrum penicillin)

Used in treatment of urinary tract infections (UTIs), asymptomatic bacteriuria, or prostatitis.

Administration

Mild infection:
Child: 30–50 mg/kg/24 hr ÷ q6h PO (max. dose: 2–3 g/24 hr)
Adult (UTI): 382–764 mg q6h PO

Nursing Implications

Use with caution in patients who are allergic to penicillin. Side effects include nausea, vomiting, diarrhea, abdominal cramps, and flatulence. May cause hepatotoxicity and furry tongue.

cefaclor (Ceclor)

Indications

(antibiotic; second-generation cephalosporin)

Used in treatment of OM; respiratory, skin, and bone and joint infections; and UTIs.

Administration

Infant or child: 20–40 mg/kg/24 hr ÷ q8h PO (max. dose: 2g/24 hr)
May give q12h in OM or pharyngitis
Adult: 250–500 mg/dose q8h PO (max. dose: 4g/24 hr)

Nursing Implications

Use with caution in children with penicillin sensitivity or impaired renal function. May cause a positive Coombs' test or a false-positive test for urinary glucose. Also can cause nausea, vomiting, diarrhea, and rash. Food or milk delays and decreases peak concentration with capsules and suspension, so give 1 hr before or 2 hr after meals.

cefazolin (Ancef, Kefzol)

Indications

(antibiotic; first-generation cephalosporin)

Used in treatment of serious skin infections; respiratory tract, urinary tract, and bone and joint infections; and septicemia. Also used as prophylactic antibiotic for invasive procedures.

Administration

Neonate:

≤7 days:	40 mg/kg/24 hr ÷ q12h IV/IM
>7 days, ≤2 kg:	40 mg/kg/24 hr ÷ q12h IV/IM
>2 kg:	60 mg/kg/24 hr ÷ q8h IV/IM
Infant >1 mo/child:	50–100 mg/kg/24 hr ÷ q8h IV/IM (max. dose: 6g/24 hr)
Adult:	2–6g/24 hr ÷ q6–8h IV/IM (max. dose: 12g/24 hr)

IV dilution:

Direct IV:	Max. concentration: 100 mg/mL over 3–5 min
Intermittent infusion:	20 mg/mL over 10–60 min
Compatibility:	D_5W, NS, LR

Nursing Implications

Use with caution in children with penicillin sensitivity or impaired renal function. May cause phlebitis, leukopenia, thrombocytopenia, transient increase in liver enzymes, false-positive urine-reducing substance, and positive Coombs' test.

cefixime (Suprax)

Indications

(antibiotic; third-generation cephalosporin)

Used in treatment of mild UTIs, OM, bronchitis, pharyngitis, and tonsillitis.

Administration

Infant or child:	8 mg/kg/24 hr ÷ q12–24 hr PO (max. dose: 400 mg/24 hr)
Adolescent or adult:	400 mg/24 hr ÷ q12–24 hr PO

Nursing Implications

Use with caution in children with penicillin sensitivity or impaired renal function. Can cause diarrhea, abdominal pain, nausea, and HA. Administer with food to decrease GI upset. Tablets not effective in treatment of OM; use suspension.

cefotaxime (Claforan)

Indications

(antibiotic; third-generation cephalosporin)

Used in treatment of skin, bone, joint, urinary, gynecologic, respiratory, and intraabdominal infections, as well as septicemia and meningitis.

Administration

Neonate:

≤7 days, <2 kg:	100 mg/kg/24 hr ÷ q12h IV/IM
≥2 kg:	100–150 mg/kg/24 hr ÷ q8–12h IV/IM
>7 days, <1.2 kg:	100 mg/kg/24 hr ÷ q12h IV/IM
≥1.2 kg:	150 mg/kg/24 hr ÷ q8h IV/IM
Infant or child (<50 kg):	100–200 mg/kg/24 hr ÷ q6–8h IV/IM
Meningitis:	200 mg/kg/24 hr ÷ q6h IV/IM (max. dose: 12 g/ 24 hr)
Adults (≥50 kg):	1–2 g/dose ÷ q6–8h IV/IM (max. dose: 12 g/ 24 hr)

IV dilution:

Direct IV:	Max. concentration: 100 mg/mL (200 mg/mL CVL) over 3–5 min
Intermittent infusion:	20–60 mg/mL over 10–30 min
Compatibility:	D_5W, NS, LR

Nursing Implications

Use with caution in children with pencillin sensitivity and in impaired renal function. Can cause neutropenia; thrombocytopenia; eosinophilia; positive Coombs' test; and transient increased blood urea nitrogen (BUN), creatinine, and liver enzymes.

cefoxitin (Mefoxin)

Indications

(antibiotic; second-generation cephalosporin)

Used in treatment of skin, bone, joint, respiratory tract, urinary tract, intraabdominal, and gynecologic infections.

Administration

Infant or child:	80–160 mg/kg/24 hr ÷ q4–8h IV/IM
Adult:	4–12 g/24 hr ÷ q6–8h IV/IM (max. dose: 12 g/24 hr)

IV dilution:

Direct IV:	Max. concentration: 100 mg/mL over 3–5 min
Intermittent infusion:	10–40 mg/mL over 10–60 min
Compatibility:	D_5W, NS, LR, $D_{10}W$

Nursing Implications

Use with caution in children with penicillin sensitivity and in impaired renal function. Can cause HA; fever; rash; pseudomembranous colitis; nausea; vomiting; diarrhea; positive direct Coombs' test; transient elevation of BUN, creatinine, and LFTs; and transient leukopenia, thrombocytopenia, neutropenia, anemia, and eosinophilia.

cefprozil (Cefzil)

Indications

(antibiotic; second-generation cephalosporin)
Used in treatment of respiratory tract and skin infections and OM.

Administration

OM: 6 mo–12 yr:	30 mg/kg/24 hr ÷ q12h PO
Pharyngitis or tonsillitis: 2–12 yr:	15 mg/kg/24 hr ÷ q12h PO
Other: ≥12 yr:	500–1,000 mg/24 hr ÷ q12–24h PO (max. dose: 1 g/24 hr)

Nursing Implications

Absorption not affected by food. Can cause HA, rash, nausea, vomiting, and serum sickness-like reactions.

ceftazidime (Fortaz, Ceptaz, Tazadime)

Indications

(antibiotic; third-generation cephalosporin)
Same as in cefoxitin, plus septicemia, meningitis, osteomyelitis, and cystic fibrosis (CF).

Administration

Neonate:

≤7 days:	100 mg/kg/24 hr ÷ q12h IV/IM
>7 days, <1.2 kg:	100 mg/kg/24 hr ÷ q12h IV/IM
≥1.2 kg:	150 mg/kg/24 hr ÷ q8h IV/IM

Infant or child:	90–150 mg/kg/24 hr ÷ q8h IV/IM
Meningitis:	150 mg/kg/24 hr ÷ q8h IV/IM
CF:	150 mg/kg/24 hr ÷ q8h IV/IM
Adult:	2–6 g/24 hr ÷ q8–12h IV/IM (max. dose: 6 g/24 hr)

IV dilution:
Direct IV:	Max. concentration: 100 mg/mL over 3–5 min
Intermittent infusion (preferred):	≤40 mg/mL over 15–30 min
Compatibility:	D$_5$W, NS, LR

Nursing Implications

See cefoxitin.

ceftriaxone (Rocephin)

Indications

(antibiotic; third-generation cephalosporin)

Used in treatment of sepsis; meningitis; lower respiratory tract infections; skin, bone, and joint infections; documented or suspected gonococcal infections; and resistant OM.

Administration

Neonate:
Gonococcal ophthalmia or prophylaxis:	25–50 mg/kg/dose × 1 IV/IM (max. dose: 125 mg/dose)
Infant or child:	50–75 mg/kg/24 hr ÷ q12–24h IV/IM
	80–100 mg/kg/24 hr ÷ q12–24h IV/IM recommended for infections outside the CSF caused by penicillin-resistant pneumococci
Meningitis:	100 mg/kg/24 hr ÷ q12h IV/IM (max. dose: 4 g/24 hr)
Acute OM:	50 mg/kg IM × 1 (max. dose: 1 g)
Adult:	1–4 g/24 hr ÷ q12–24h IV/IM (max. dose: 4 g/24 hr)
Gonococcal prophylaxis or uncomplicated gonorrhea:	125 mg IM × 1 dose
Chancroid:	250 mg IM × 1 dose

IV dilution:
Direct IV:	Max. concentration: 40 mg/mL over 3–5 min

Intermittent infusion
(preferred):   10–40 mg/mL over 10–30 min
Compatibility: D$_5$W, NS, LR, D$_{10}$W

Nursing Implications

Use with caution in children with penicillin sensitivity or impaired renal
function. May cause jaundice, reversible cholelithiasis, HA, nausea, vomiting, and diarrhea.

cefuroxime, cefuroxime axetil (Zinacef IV/IM, Ceftin PO)

Indications

(antibiotic; second-generation cephalosporin)
   Used same as other cephalosporins. Not recommended for meningitis.
PO form used to treat OM, pharyngitis, tonsillitis, and impetigo.

Administration

Neonate: 20–60 mg/kg/24 hr ÷ q12h IV/IM
Infant or child: 75–100 mg/kg/24 hr ÷ q8h IV/IM (max. dose:
                               6 g/24 hr)

Pharyngitis:
   Suspension: 20 mg/kg/24 hr ÷ q12h PO (max. dose: 500 mg/
                               24 hr)
   Tablet: 125 mg q12h
OM or impetigo:
   Suspension: 30 mg/kg/24 hr ÷ q12h PO (max. dose: 1 g/24 hr)
   Tablet: 250 mg q12h
Adult: 750 mg–1.5 g/dose q8h IV/IM (max. dose: 9 g/
                               24 hr)
                             250–500 mg b.i.d. PO (max. dose: 1 g/24 hr)

IV dilution:
   Direct IV: Max. concentration: 100 mg/mL over 3–5 min
   Intermittent infusion
   (preferred):   ≤30 mg/mL over 15–30 min
Compatibility: D$_5$W, NS, LR, D$_{10}$W

Nursing Implications

Use with caution in children with penicillin sensitivity or impaired renal
function. May cause thrombophlebitis at infusion site. Tablets and suspension are not equivalent and cannot be substituted on a mg-to-mg basis.
Administer suspension with food. Most common side effects are HA, rash,
nausea, vomiting, and diarrhea.

cephalexin (Keflex)

Indications

(antibiotic; first-generation cephalosporin)

Used to treat skin infections including impetigo; group A beta hemolytic streptococcal infections; OM; and infections of the respiratory tract, bone, and GU tract.

Administration

Infant or child: 25–100 mg/kg/24 hr ÷ q6–12h PO
Adult: 1–4 g/24 hr ÷ q6–12h PO (max. dose: 4 g/24 hr)

Nursing Implications

Use with caution in children with penicillin sensitivity and in impaired renal function. Can cause GI disturbance, HA, and rash. Absorbed best on an empty stomach but can be given with food or milk to decrease GI irritation. Less frequent dosing such as q8–12h can be used for uncomplicated infections.

cephalothin (Keflin)

Indications

(antibiotic; first-generation cephalosporin)

Used to treat respiratory tract, skin, urinary tract, bone, and joint infections; endocarditis; and septicemia.

Administration

Neonate:

≤7 days, <2 kg:	40 mg/kg/24 hr ÷ q12h IV
≥2 kg:	60 mg/kg/24 hr ÷ q8h IV
>7 days, <2 kg:	40–60 mg/kg/24 hr ÷ q8–12h IV
≥2 kg:	80 mg/kg/24 hr ÷ q6h IV
Infant or child:	80–160 mg/kg/24 hr ÷ q4–6h IV or deep IM
Adult:	2–12 g/24 hr ÷ q4–6h IV/IM (max. dose: 12 g/ 24 hr)

IV dilution:

Direct IV:	Max. concentration: 100 mg/mL over 3–5 min
Intermittent infusion:	≤100 mg/mL over 30–60 min
Compatibility:	D₅W, NS, LR, SW

Nursing Implications

Can cause HA, rash, nausea, vomiting, diarrhea, and severe phlebitis, especially with doses >6 g/24 hr for >3 days.

cetirizine (Zyrtec)

Indications

(antihistamine, less sedating)
   Used in perennial and seasonal allergic rhinitis and in chronic idiopathic urticaria.

Administration

Child 2–5 yr: Initial dose 2.5 mg daily PO, if needed can increase dose to max. dose of 5 mg/24 hr PO
≥6 yr–adult: 5–10 mg daily PO

Nursing Implications

May cause HA, pharyngitis, GI symptoms, dry mouth, and sedation. Give dose at bedtime if sedation is a problem.

charcoal (Actidose, CharcoAid, Liqui-Char)

Indications

(antidote)
   Used as an emergency antidote in treatment of poisoning.

Administration

Acute poisoning single dose: 1–2 g/kg up to 15–30 g PO
Acute poisoning multiple doses: 1–2 g/kg PO q4–6 hours

Nursing Implications

Usually available as premixed solutions. Solutions containing sorbitol should not be used for multiple doses because diarrhea will occur. Not to be administered at the same time as ipecac because charcoal will absorb and inactivate the ipecac. Do not administer with dairy products because absorption of charcoal will be decreased. Side effects include GI discomfort, diarrhea, and intestinal gas.

chloral hydrate (Noctec)

Indications

(sedative; hypnotic)
   Used for short-term sedation and before procedures.

Administration

Child:
   Sedative: 25–50 mg/kg/24 hr q6–8h PO/PR (max. dose: 500 mg)

Procedure: 25–100 mg/kg/dose PO/PR (max. dose: infant–1 g;
child–2 g)
Adult:
Sedative: 250 mg/dose t.i.d. PO/PR
Hypnotic: 500–1,000 mg/dose PO/PR (max. dose: 2 g/24 hr)

Nursing Implications

Irritating to mucous membranes. Can cause GI irritation, paradoxic excitement, hypotension, and heart and respiratory depression. Can accumulate
with repeated use. Do not use in children with liver or renal impairment.
Use with caution in children with heart disease or those on furosemide (IV)
or anticoagulants. Peak effects in 30–60 min. Do not exceed 2 wk of
chronic use. Sudden withdrawal can cause delirium tremens.

chloramphenicol (Chloromycetin)

Indications

(antibiotic)

Used in treatment of serious skin and soft tissue, intraabdominal, and
CNS infections and bacteremia when organisms are resistant to other less
toxic antibiotics. Also used in treatment of rickettsial infections such as
Rocky Mountain spotted fever and typhus. Topical and ophthalmic routes
are used for local management of superficial infections.

Administration

Ophthalmic: 1–2 gtt. or ribbon of ointment in each eye
q3–6h

Topical: Apply to affected area t.i.d.–q.i.d.
Neonate:
Loading dose: 20 mg/kg IV
Maintenance dose:
≤7 days: 25 mg/kg/24 hr daily IV
>7 days, ≤2 kg: 25 mg/kg/24 hr daily IV
>2 kg: 50 mg/kg/24 hr ÷ q12h IV
First maintenance dose should be given 12 hr after loading dose.
Infant, child, or adult: 50–75 mg/kg/24 hr IV/PO ÷ q6h
Meningitis: 75–100 mg/kg/24 hr ÷ q6h IV (max. dose: 4 g/
24 hr)

IV dilution:
Direct IV: Max. concentration: 100 mg/mL over 5 min
Intermittent infusion: ≤20 mg/mL over 15–30 min
Compatibility: D$_5$W, NS, LR

Nursing Implications

Monitor blood levels. Therapeutic levels: 15–25 mg/L for meningitis; 10–20 mg/L for other infections. PO doses achieve higher levels than IV doses. Use with caution in G6PD deficiency, in renal or hepatic dysfunction, and in neonates. Can cause three major toxicities: bone marrow suppression; gray syndrome of the newborn, characterized by circulatory collapse, hypothermia, coma, and death; and aplastic anemia 3 wk to 12 mo after initial exposure to chloramphenicol. Also can cause HA, rash, diarrhea, vomiting, and anaphylaxis. Because of the major toxicities after both short- and long-term use, chloramphenicol is not used when less toxic agents are effective.

cimetidine (Tagamet)

Indications

(histamine-2 antagonist)

Used for short-term treatment and long-term prophylaxis of duodenal ulcers; treatment of benign gastric ulcers; management of GE reflux; and to inhibit gastric acid secretion.

Administration

Neonate:	5–20 mg/kg/24 hr ÷ q6–12h PO/IV/IM
Infant:	10–20 mg/kg/24 hr ÷ q6h PO/IV/IM
Child:	20–40 mg/kg/24 hr ÷ q6h PO/IV/IM
Adult:	300 mg/dose q.i.d., 400 mg/dose b.i.d., *or* 800 mg/dose q.h.s. PO/IV/IM
Ulcer prophylaxis:	400–800 mg q.h.s. PO (max. dose: 2,400 mg/ 24 hr)
IV dilution:	
Direct IV:	Max. concentration: 15 mg/mL over 15 min
Intermittent infusion (preferred):	6 mg/mL over 15–30 min
Compatibility:	D_5W, NS, LR, $D_{10}W$

Nursing Implications

Rapid IV administration can cause hypotension, arrhythmias, cardiac arrest. Also can cause rash, mild diarrhea, nausea and vomiting, myalgia, neutropenia, gynecomastia, elevated LFTs, and dizziness. Do not give PO with antacids.

ciprofloxacin (Cipro, Ciloxan ophthalmic, Cipro HC otic)

Indications

(antibiotic; quinolone)

Used in treatment of documented or suspected pseudomonal or serious drug-resistant infections of the respiratory or urinary tract, skin, bone, joint, eye, and ear.

Administration

Child: 20–30 mg/kg/24 hr ÷ q12h PO (max. dose: 1.5 g/24 hr)
              10–20 mg/kg/24 hr ÷ q12h IV (max. dose: 800 mg/24 hr)
CF: 40 mg/kg/24 hr ÷ q12h PO (max. dose: 2 g/24 hr)
              30 mg/kg/24 hr ÷ q8h IV (max. dose: 1.2 g/24 hr)
Adult: 250–750 mg/dose q12h PO
              200–400 mg/dose q12h IV
Ophthalmic: 1–2 gtt. q2h while awake × 2 days, then 1–2 gtt. q4h while awake × 5 days
Otic (>1 yr) or
   adult: 3 gtt. to affected ear b.i.d. × 7 days
IV dilution: Not to exceed max. concentration: 2 mg/mL over 60 min
Compatibility: D_5W, NS

Nursing Implications

Can cause GI upset, renal failure. GI symptoms, HA, restlessness, and rash are most common side effects. Use with caution in children <18 years. Can increase effect or toxicity of theophylline, warfarin, and cyclosporin. Do not administer antacids with or within 2–4 hr after PO ciprofloxacin dose. Shake suspension vigorously before administration. IV administration given too quickly can cause swelling, pain, burning, and phlebitis.

clarithromycin (Biaxin)

Indications

(antibiotic; macrolide)

Used in treatment of upper and lower respiratory tract infections, acute OM, and infections of the skin and skin structures, as well as for prophylaxis and treatment of *Mycobacterium avium* complex (MAC) disease in patients with advanced HIV infection, treatment of *Helicobacter pylori* infection, and prophylaxis of bacterial endocarditis in patients who are allergic to penicillin.

Administration

Child:
   OM, pharyngitis, pneumonia,
      sinusitis, skin infection: 15 mg/kg/24 hr ÷ q12h PO
   MAC prophylaxis: 15 mg/kg/24 hr ÷ q12h PO

Bacterial endocarditis prophylaxis:	15 mg/kg 1 hr before procedure (max. dose: 1 g/24 hr)
Adult:	250–500 mg/dose q12h PO
MAC prophylaxis:	500 mg/dose q12h PO
Bacterial endocarditis prophylaxis:	500 mg 1 hr before procedure

Nursing Implications

Contraindicated in patients allergic to erythromycin. May cause diarrhea, nausea, abnormal taste, dyspepsia, abdominal discomfort, and HA. May increase carbamazepine, theophylline, and cyclosporin levels. May be administered with food.

clindamycin (Cleocin)

Indications

(antibiotic)

Used in treatment of skin, respiratory tract, intraabdominal, and gynecologic infections; septicemia; and osteomyelitis. Topical used in treatment of severe acne.

Administration

Neonate:	
≤7 days, ≤2 kg:	5 mg/kg/dose ÷ q12h IV/IM
>2 kg:	5 mg/kg/dose ÷ q8h IV/IM
>7 days, <1.2 kg:	5 mg/kg/dose ÷ q12h IV/IM
1.2–2 kg:	5 mg/kg/dose ÷ q8h IV/IM
>2 kg:	5 mg/kg/dose ÷ q6h IV/IM
Child:	10–30 mg/kg/24 hr ÷ q6–8h PO
	25–40 mg/kg/24 hr ÷ q6–8h IV/IM
Adult:	150–450 mg/dose q6–8h PO (max. dose: 1.8 g/ 24 hr)
	1,200–1,800 mg/24 hr ÷ q6–12h IV/IM (max. dose: 4.8 g/24 hr)
Topical:	Apply to affected area b.i.d.
IV dilution:	Max. concentration: 18 mg/mL over 10–60 min
	Do not exceed 30 mg/min
Compatibility:	D₅W, NS, LR

Nursing Implications

Contraindicated in liver impairment and diarrhea. Can cause diarrhea, rash. Rapid infusion can cause cardiac arrest. Not indicated in meningitis.

Pseudomembranous colitis may occur up to several weeks after stopping drug. Can also cause Stevens-Johnson syndrome, granulocytopenia, thrombocytopenia, or sterile abscess at injection site.

clonidine (Catapres)

Indications

(antihypertensive; central α-adrenergic agonist)
Used in management of hypertension and as alternate agent for treatment of attention deficit hyperactivity disorder (ADHD).

Administration

Child: 5–7 μg/kg/24 hr ÷ q6–12h PO; increase to 5–25 μg/kg/24 hr at 5- to 7-day intervals as needed (max. dose: 0.9 mg/24 hr)
Adult: 0.1 mg b.i.d. PO initially; increase in 0.1-mg/24 hr increments at weekly intervals until desired response is achieved (max. dose: 2.4 mg/24 hr)

Nursing Implications

OK to give with food. Side effects include dry mouth, dizziness, drowsiness, fatigue, constipation, anorexia, arrhythmias, and hypotension. Must be tapered gradually over 1 wk to discontinue.

clotrimazole (Lotrimin, Mycelex)

Indications

(antifungal)
Used to treat fungal infections of the mouth, skin, and vulvovaginal area.

Administration

Topical:	Apply to skin b.i.d. × 4–8 wk
Vaginal candidiasis (vaginal tabs):	100 mg/dose q.h.s. × 7 days
	200 mg/dose q.h.s. × 3 days *or*
	500 mg/dose × 1 *or*
	1 applicator dose (5 g) of 1% vaginal cream q.h.s. × 7–10 days
>3 yr–adult: Thrush:	Slowly dissolve one 10-mg troche in mouth 5x/24 hr × 14 days

Nursing Implications

May cause erythema, blistering, or urticaria with topical use. Also can increase liver enzymes and cause nausea and vomiting when given orally.

codeine (Many brands)

Indications

(narcotic; analgesic; antitussive)
Used to treat mild to moderate pain. Used as an antitussive in smaller doses.

Administration

Analgesic:

Child:	0.5–1 mg/kg/dose q4–6h PO/IM/SC (max. dose: 60 mg/dose)
Adult:	15–60 mg/dose q4–6h PO/IM/SC
Tylenol with Codeine:	Elixir contains acetaminophen 120 mg and codeine 12 mg/5 mL (7% alcohol)
	Tablets with codeine contain 300 mg acetaminophen/tablet
Tylenol #1:	7.5 mg codeine
Tylenol #2:	15 mg codeine
Tylenol #3:	30 mg codeine
Tylenol #4:	60 mg codeine
Antitussive:	All doses p.r.n.; 1–1.5 mg/kg/24 hr ÷ q4–6h; alternatively dose by age as follows:
Child 2–6 yr:	2.5–5 mg/dose q4–6h PO (max. dose: 30 mg/24 hr)
Child 6–12 yr:	5–10 mg/dose q4–6h PO (max. dose: 60 mg/24 hr)
Adult:	10–20 mg/dose q4–6h PO (max. dose: 120 mg/24 hr)

Nursing Implications

Observe for excessive sedation and respiratory depression. Can also cause nausea, constipation, cramping, hypotension, and pruritus. For best pain-relief effects, use with acetaminophen. Do not use as an antitussive in children <2 yr. Give with food to decrease nausea and GI upset. Can be habit forming. *Do not give IV.*

cotrimoxazole (Bactrim, Septra, Cotrim)

Indications

(antibiotic; sulfonamide derivative)
Used in treatment of bronchitis, shigellosis, typhoid fever, OM, and diarrhea. Used for prophylaxis and treatment of *Pneumocystis carinii* pneumonia (PCP) and UTIs.

Administration

Doses based on trimethoprim (TMP) component:
Minor infections:

Child:	8–10 mg/kg/24 hr ÷ b.i.d. IV/PO
Adult (>40 kg):	160 mg/dose b.i.d.
UTI prophylaxis:	2–4 mg/kg/24 hr daily
Severe infections and PCP:	20 mg/kg/24 hr ÷ q6–8h IV/PO
PCP prophylaxis:	5–10 mg/kg/24 hr ÷ b.i.d. 3 consecutive days/wk (max. dose: 320 mg/24 hr)
IV dilution:	1:25 (5 mL of drug to 125 mL of IV fluid) over 60–90 min
	Do not give direct IV
Compatibility:	D_5W, LR

Nursing Implications

Use cautiously with impaired renal or liver function. Not recommended in infants <2 mo. May cause blood dyscrasias, crystalluria, glossitis, renal or hepatic injury, GI irritation, rash, and Stevens-Johnson syndrome. Can cause hemolysis in patients with G6PD.

cromolyn (Intal, Nasalcrom, Gastrocrom, Crolom)

Indications

(antiallergic agent)

Used as oral inhalation or nebulization prophylactic agent for long-term control of persistent asthma and prevention of allergen- or exercise-induced bronchospasm. Used intranasally to manage seasonal or perennial allergic rhinitis. Ophthalmic used to treat vernal conjunctivitis. Oral route used to treat systemic mastocytosis, food allergy, and inflammatory bowel disease (IBD).

Administration

Spin inhalant:	20 mg q6–8h
Nebulization:	20 mg q6–8h
Nasal:	1 spray each nostril t.i.d.–q.i.d.
MDI:	
Child:	1–2 puffs t.i.d.–q.i.d.
Adult:	2–4 puffs t.i.d.–q.i.d.
Ophthalmic:	1–2 gtt. 4–6x/24 hr
Food allergy or IBD:	
Child >2 yr:	100 mg q.i.d. PO; give 15–20 min a.c. and q.h.s. (max. dose: 40 mg/kg/24 hr)
Adult:	200–400 mg q.i.d. PO; give 15–20 min a.c. and q.h.s.

Systemic mastocytosis:

<2 yr:	20 mg/kg/24 hr ÷ q.i.d. PO (max. dose: 30 mg/kg/24 hr)
2–12 yr:	100 mg q.i.d. PO (max. dose: 40 mg/kg/24 hr)
Adult:	200 mg q.i.d. PO

Nursing Implications

Can cause rash, bronchospasm, cough, and nasal congestion. Oral use can cause HA and diarrhea. Therapeutic response occurs within 2 wk, but may take 4–6 wk to determine maximum benefit. For exercise-induced bronchospasm, give not longer than 1 hr before exercise. Nebulizer solution can be mixed with albuterol.

cyclosporine (Sandimmune)
Indications

(immunosuppressant)
Used to prevent organ rejection of kidney, liver, and heart.

Administration

PO:	Initially, 15 mg/kg single dose 4–12 hr prior to transplantation
	Continue daily dose of 10–14 mg/kg/day for 1–2 weeks tapered by 5%/wk over 6–8 weeks
	Maintenance dose: 5–10 mg/kg/day
IV:	Initially, 5–6 mg/kg single dose 4–12 hr prior to transplantation
	Continue this daily single dose until patient is able to take PO dosage
IV dilution:	Dilute each mL concentrate with 20–100 mL compatible fluid. Infuse over 2–6 hours, monitoring patient continuously for first 30 minutes for signs of hypersensitivity.
Compatibility:	D$_5$W, 0.9% NaCl

Nursing Implications

Oral solution may be mixed in *glass* container with milk, chocolate milk, or orange juice. Side effects include mild to moderate hypertension, hirsutism, and tremor. Grapefruit and grapefruit juice should be avoided because these increase the side effects of the medication. To monitor for nephrotoxicity and hepatotoxicity, monitor BUN, creatinine, and LFTs. Diligent oral care is necessary to prevent gum hyperplasia. Therapeutic blood serum level: 50–300 ng/mL.

deferoxamine mesylate (Desferal)

Indications

(chelating agent)

Used to treat acute iron poisoning and chronic iron overload in children receiving chronic blood transfusions.

Administration

Acute iron poisoning:

Child:	15 mg/kg/hr IV
	50 mg/kg/dose q6h IM (max. dose: 6 g/24 hr)
Adult:	15 mg/kg/hr IV
	1 g × 1, then 0.5 g q4–12h IM (max. dose: 6 g/ 24 hr)

Chronic iron overload:

Child:	15 mg/kg/hr IV
	20–40 mg/kg/dose daily as infusion over 8–12 hr SC
Adult:	0.5–1 g/dose daily IM
	1–2 g/dose as infusion over 8–24 hr SC
IV dilution:	Max. concentration: 250 mg/mL
	Max. rate: 15 mg/kg/hr
Compatibility:	D_5W, NS, LR

Nursing Implications

Contraindicated in anuria. May cause flushing, erythema, urticaria, hypotension, tachycardia, diarrhea, leg cramps, fever, cataracts, and hearing loss. SC not recommended for acute iron poisoning. May cause urine to turn reddish color. Rotate SC sites. Painful lumps with SC administration may indicate rate too fast or needle too close to skin.

desmopressin acetate (DDAVP) (DDAVP, Stimate)

Indications

(vasopressin analog, synthetic; hemostatic agent)

Used in treatment of diabetes insipidus, to control bleeding in certain types of hemophilia, and for primary nocturnal enuresis (bedwetting).

Administration

Diabetes insipidus:

Child:	0.05 mg b.i.d. PO; titrate to effect
3 mo–12 yr:	5–30 µg/24 hr ÷ daily–b.i.d. intranasally

Adult:	0.05 mg b.i.d. PO; titrate to effect, range 0.1–0.2 mg/24 hr ÷ b.i.d.–t.i.d.
	10–40 μg/24 hr ÷ daily–t.i.d. intranasally; titrate to achieve control of thirst and urination (max. intranasal dose: 40 μg/ 24 hr)
IV/SC:	2–4 μg/24 hr ÷ b.i.d.
Hemophilia A and von Willebrand's disease:	
Intranasal:	2–4 μg/kg/dose (give 2 hr before procedure)
IV:	0.2–0.4 μg/kg/dose over 15–30 min (give 30 min before procedure)
Nocturnal enuresis (>6 yr):	
PO:	0.2 mg h.s.; titrated to 0.6 mg to achieve desired effect
Intranasal:	20 μg h.s.; range 10–40 μg; divide dose by 2 and put each half dose per nostril
IV dilution:	0.5 μg/mL over 15–30 min
Compatibility:	NS only

Nursing Implications

May cause HA, nausea, hyponatremia, nasal congestion, abdominal cramps, and hypertension. Stimate spray pump must be primed before first use; discard after 25 doses; further doses may be subpotent. Avoid using spray in children <6 yr because of difficulty in titrating dosage.

dexamethasone (Decadron and others)

Implications

(corticosteroid)

Used to manage allergic, inflammatory, hematologic, neoplastic, and autoimmune disorders. Also used in management of cerebral edema and septic shock, as well as before or with first dose of antibiotic in meningitis.

Administration

Cerebral edema:	
Loading dose:	1–2 mg/kg/dose PO/IV/IM × 1
Maintenance:	1–1.5 mg/kg/24 hr ÷ q4–6h PO/IV/IM (max. dose: 16 mg/24 hr)
Airway edema:	0.5–2 mg/kg/24 hr ÷ q6h PO/IV/IM
Croup:	0.6 mg/kg/dose × 1 IV/IM

Antiemetic (chemotherapy
    induced):
    Initial: 10 mg/m^2/dose IV (max. dose: 20 mg)
    Subsequent: 5 mg/m^2/dose ÷ q6h IV
Anti-inflammatory:
    Child: 0.08–0.3 mg/kg/24 hr ÷ q6–12h PO/IV/IM
    Adult: 0.75–9 mg/24 hr ÷ q6–12h PO/IV/IM
Meningitis (>6 wk):   0.6 mg/kg/24 hr ÷ q6h IV × 2 days
IV dilution:
    Direct IV: 4 mg/mL over 1–4 min for doses <10 mg
    Intermittent IV: 1 mg/mL over 15–30 min
Compatibility: D$_5$W, NS, LR

Nursing Implications

Can cause hypertension, HA, pseudotumor cerebri, adrenal suppression,
nausea, vomiting, Cushing's syndrome, muscle weakness, and osteoporosis.
May give with food to decrease GI symptoms.

dextroamphetamine (Biphetamine, Dexedrine, Ferdex, Oxydess II)

Indications

(CNS stimulant)
    Used to treat ADHD and narcolepsy and for obesity control (in chil-
dren >12 yr).

Administration

ADHD:
    3–5 yr: 2.5 mg/24 hr q AM PO; increase by 2.5 mg/24 hr at
                              weekly intervals (max. dose: 40 mg/24 hr)
    ≥6 yr: 5 mg/24 hr
Obesity (>12 yr):   5–30 mg/24 hr PO in divided doses of 10–15 mg taken
                              30–60 min before meals *or* 10- to 15-mg extended-
                              release capsule q AM
Narcolepsy:
    6–12 yr: 5 mg/24 hr PO initially; may increase at 5-mg
                              increments q wk until side effects appear (max.
                              dose: 60 mg/day)
    >12 yr–adult: 10 mg/24 hr PO initially; may increase at 10-mg
                              increments q wk until side effects appear (max.
                              dose: 60 mg/day)

Nursing Implications

Classified as schedule-II drug under Federal Controlled Substances Act. Monitor pulse and BP. For children with ADHD, obtain caregiver and teacher report about behavioral performance. Many side effects, including insomnia, HA, vomiting, abdominal cramps, restlessness, anorexia, psychosis, dry mouth, and growth failure.

diazepam (Valium and others)

Indications

(anticonvulsant; anxiolytic, benzodiazepine)

Used in management of general anxiety disorders, for sedation, to treat status epilepticus, and as a muscle relaxant.

Administration

Sedative or muscle
   relaxant:

Child:	0.04–0.2 mg/kg/dose q2–4h IV/IM (max. dose: 0.6 mg/kg in 8 hr)
	0.12–0.8 mg/kg/24 hr ÷ q6–8h PO
Adult:	2–10 mg/dose q3–4h p.r.n. IV/IM
	2–20 mg/dose q6–12h p.r.n. PO

Status epilepticus:

Neonate:	0.3–0.75 mg/kg/dose q15–30 min IV × 2–3 doses
>1 mo:	0.2–0.5 mg/kg/dose q15–30 min IV (max. total dose: <5 yr: 5 mg; ≥5 yr: 10 mg)
IV dilution:	Give undiluted push over 3 min (max. dose: 2 mg/min)

Compatibility: Do not mix with any IV fluids; administer as close to site as possible because it interacts with the plastic IV tubing.

Nursing Implications

Hypotension and respiratory depression can occur. CNS depressants, cimetidine, erythromycin, and valproic acid may enhance effects of diazepam.

dicloxacillin (Dynapen, Pathocil, and others)

Indications

(antibiotic; penicillin, penicillinase-resistant)

Used in treatment of skin and soft-tissue infections and pneumonia and as follow-up therapy for osteomyelitis.

Administration

Child (<40 kg):

Mild to moderate infections:	12.5–25 mg/kg/24 hr ÷ q6h PO
Severe infections:	50–100 mg/kg/24 hr ÷ q6h PO
Adult (≥40 kg):	125–500 mg/dose q6h PO (max. dose: 4 g/24 hr)

Nursing Implications

Administer 1–2 hr before or 2 hr after meals. Can cause nausea, vomiting, and diarrhea.

digoxin (Lanoxin)

Implications

(antiarrhythmic agent; inotrope)

Used in treatment of CHF to slow HR in atrial fibrillation and flutter and to end paroxysmal atrial tachycardia. Increases force of myocardial contraction; decreases conduction through sinoatrial (SA) and atrioventricular (AV) nodes. Increases cardiac output.

Administration

Maintenance doses:

Neonate (full term):	8–10 μg/kg/24 hr b.i.d. PO
	6–8 μg/kg/24 hr b.i.d. IV/IM
Child <2 yr:	10–12 μg/kg/24 hr b.i.d. PO
	7.5–9 μg/kg/24 hr b.i.d. IV/IM
2–10 yr:	8–10 μg/kg/24 hr b.i.d. PO
	6–8 μg/kg/24 hr b.i.d. IV/IM
>10 yr (<100 kg):	2.5–5 μg/kg/24 hr daily PO
	2–3 μg/kg/24 hr daily IV/IM
IV dilution:	Undiluted or diluted at least 4-fold slowly over 5–10 min
	Max. concentration: Child: 100 μg/mL; adult: 250 μg/mL
Compatibility:	D_5W, NS, $D_{10}W$

Nursing Implications

Children started on digoxin are given total digitalizing dose (TDD), which is approximately 4 × maintenance dose initially, as follows: 1/2 the TDD, then 1/4 the TDD q8–18h × 2, then ECG is obtained to assess for toxicity. If tolerated, client is started on maintenance dose as listed previously. Check apical pulse for 1 full min before administration. Hold dose and check with doctor if HR <90–100 bpm for an infant, 70 bpm for a child, and 60 bpm for an adult, or according to hospital policy. IV dose should be double-checked before administering. Less than 4-fold dilution can cause precipitation. Therapeutic levels: 0.8–2.0 ng/mL. Most common side effects in infants and children are nausea and vomiting. IM route usually not recommended because of local irritation, pain, and tissue damage.

dimercaprol (BAL in oil)

Indications

(antidote; chelating agent)
Used in the treatment of acute lead poisoning.

Administration

Severe poisoning: 4 mg/kg by deep IM injection then q4h for 2–7 days. For less severe poisoning, dosage is 3 mg/kg after the first dose.

Nursing Implications

Rotate the sites of IM injection. Don't let medication come in contact with skin because it can cause a skin reaction. For acute lead encephalopathy, given in combination with edetate calcium disodium but in different IM injection sites. Renal toxicity can be minimized by keeping urine alkaline. *Do not give IV.* Drug has unpleasant garlic-type odor.

diphenhydramine (Benadryl)

Indications

(antihistamine)
Used in treatment of allergic symptoms caused by histamine release such as nasal allergies and allergic dermatosis, for mild nighttime sedation, for motion-sickness prevention, and as an antitussive. Also used in anaphylaxis and phenothiazine overdose (OD).

Administration

Child:	5 mg/kg/24 hr ÷ q6h PO/IV/IM (max. dose: 300 mg/24 hr)
Adult:	10–50 mg/dose q4–8h PO/IV/IM (max. dose: 400 mg/24 hr)
Anaphylaxis/phenothiazine OD:	1–2 mg/kg IV
IV dilution:	Max. concentration: 25 mg/mL over 10–15 min
	Max. rate: 25 mg/min
Compatibility:	D$_5$W, NS, LR

Nursing Implications

Contraindicated in acute asthma. Use cautiously in liver impairment. Can cause drowsiness, dizziness, and dry mouth. May cause paradoxical excitement in children.

divalproex sodium (Depakote)

Indications

(anticonvulsant)

See valproic acid (page 162) for indications, administration, and nursing implications. Preferred over valproic acid for patients on ketogenic diet.

docusate sodium (Colace, Senokot-S, and others)

Indications

(stool softener; laxative)

Used in patients who should avoid straining during defecation; in constipation associated with hard, dry stools; and to soften ear wax.

Administration

<3 yr:	10–40 mg/24 hr ÷ daily–q.i.d. PO
3–6 yr:	20–60 mg/24 hr ÷ daily–q.i.d. PO
6–12 yr:	40–150 mg/24 hr ÷ daily–q.i.d. PO
>12 yr:	50–500 mg/24 hr ÷ daily–q.i.d. PO
Rectal (older children or adults):	Add 50–100 mg oral solution to enema fluid
Ear:	Use a few drops of 10-mg/mL solution in ear canal to soften wax

Nursing Implications

Prolonged use leads to dependence. Oral dose may take 1–3 days of therapy to be effective. Oral solution better tolerated with milk or fruit juice.

dopamine hydrochloride (Dopastat, Intropin)

Indications

(adrenergic agonist; vasopressor)

Used to treat shock and correct hemodynamics. Improves perfusion to vital organs and increases cardiac output and BP.

Administration

Children and neonates: 1–20 mcg/kg/min IV
IV dilution: Available prediluted in 250 or 500 mL D$_5$W
Compatibility: 0.9% NaCl, D$_5$W, LR

Nursing Implications

Dosage titrated to hemodynamically desired response. Patient must be on continuous cardiac monitoring. Dopamine is most effective in patients who are not hypovolemic. Should be administered into large vein (antecubital fossa or central line) to prevent extravasation. Side effects include headache, ectopic beats, tachycardia, palpitations, nausea, and vomiting.

edetate calcium disodium (calcium EDTA)

Indications

(chelating agent)
Reduce blood levels and stores of iron in patients with lead poisoning and lead encephalopathy.

Administration

Mild to moderate lead poisoning: 25–50 mg/kg IV for 5 days
Severe lead poisoning: Up to 75 mg/kg/24 hours not to exceed 1.5 g/day

Asymptomatic lead toxicity:
  Initial: Up to 1 g/m^2/24 hr in continuous IV drip
  Subsequent courses: Up to 50 mg/kg/24 hr in continuous IV drip

Symptomatic lead toxicity:
  Initial: Up to 1.5 m/m^2/24 hr in continuous IV drip
  Subsequent courses: Up to 50 mg/kg/24 hr in continuous IV drip

Nursing Implications

Ensure hydration prior to and during administration to reduce change of treatment induced nephrotoxicity. Drug is contraindicated in cases of oliguria or anuria. Cardiac monitoring including EKG assessments should be conducted during IV administration to detect rhythm abnormalities. Intermittent doses require slow IV administration over a minimum of 4 hours to prevent encephalopathy. May be used in combination with dimercaprol (BAL) in children with lead levels higher than 70 mcg/dl.

ELA-*Max* (lidocaine 4%)

Indications

(topical analgesic)

Used as topical anesthetic on normal, intact skin for dermal anesthesia before painful procedures. May also be used for temporary relief of pain associated with minor cuts and abrasions of skin; minor burns, including sunburn; minor skin irritation; and insect bites. Is a 4% lidocaine cream in a liposomal vehicle. Liposomal encapsulation uses lipid bilayers to deliver anesthetic into dermis.

Administration

For topical use only. Thick layer of ELA-*Max* cream is applied to intact skin. Recommended application time is 15–45 min, with no occlusive dressing required.

Maximum areas for
  application in children:
  ≤10 kg: 100 cm^2 (4 × 4 in.)
  10–20 kg: 600 cm^2 (10 × 10 in.)

Nursing Implications

Explain to child that ELA-*Max* is like a "magic cream that takes hurt away."

Cream is contraindicated in areas where drug could migrate into ears or eyes and on nonintact skin.

EMLA (eutectic mixture of lidocaine 2.5% and prilocaine 2.5%)

Indications

(topical analgesic)

Used as topical anesthetic on normal, intact skin for local anesthesia before painful procedures such as IV insertion, lumbar puncture, implanted port access, peripherally inserted central catheter (PICC) line insertion, superficial biopsy, pacing wire removal, bone marrow aspiration, and IM/SC injections. As of March 11, 1999, U.S. Food and Drug Administration (FDA) has approved use of EMLA for infants born at 37 weeks' gestational age. In infants, EMLA has been safely used for newborn circumcision, IM injections of vitamin K and hepatitis B vaccine, and heel lancing for genetic testing or bilirubin levels.

Administration

For topical use only. Apply thick layer of cream to intact skin. Cover with transparent occlusive dressing (such as Tegaderm). Cream should remain as dollop. Leave in place 1 hr for minor procedures (i.e., superficial punctures) and 2 hr for major procedures (i.e., deep penetration). After removing dressing, wipe cream from skin. Test skin sensitivity and reapply if necessary. In addition to EMLA cream, the EMLA Anesthetic Disc is available, which contains 1 g of EMLA emulsion. The peel-and-stick disc is excellent for home use to anesthetize small areas (2-in. diameter).

Maximum areas for
  application in children:

<5 kg:	10 cm^2 (1.25 × 1.25 in.)
5–10 kg:	100 cm^2 (4 × 4 in.)
10–20 kg:	600 cm^2 (10 × 10 in.)
>20 kg:	2,000 cm^2 (18 × 18 in.)

Nursing Implications

Explain to child that EMLA is like a "magic cream that takes hurt away." Cream is contraindicated in areas where drug could migrate into eyes or ears, on nonintact skin or mucous membranes, in congenital or idiopathic methemoglobinemia, and in children receiving methemoglobinemia-inducing agents. Methemoglobin is a dysfunctional form of hemoglobin resulting in reduced oxygen-carrying capacity of blood and leading to cyanosis and hypoxemia. No cases of this complication have been reported in children taking acetaminophen and using EMLA. In fact, there is no evidence that acetaminophen is a methemoglobinemia-inducing drug in humans.

enoxaparin (Lovenox)

Indications

(anticoagulant; low molecular weight heparin)
  Used to prevent or treat deep vein thrombosis (DVT).

Administration

Prophylaxis:	0.5 mg/kg SQ q12h
Treatment:	1 mg/kg SQ q12h

Nursing Implications

Monitor site for hematoma. Side effects include nausea and peripheral edema. Monitor CBC, platelet count, and stool for occult blood while assessing for any sign of bleeding. Usual length of therapy is 7–10 days.

epinephrine (Adrenaline, Vaponefrin)

Indications

(adrenergic agonist; sympathomimetic; bronchodilator)
  Use to treat acute bronchial asthma attacks and hypersensitivity reactions. Restores cardiac rhythm in cardiac arrest.

Administration

Severe anaphylaxis or asthma: 0.01 mg/kg SQ (1:1,000 concentration solution)

Maximum single dose: 0.5 mg

Dose may be repeated at 20 min–4 hr intervals

Severe anaphylactic shock: 0.1 mg IV (10 mL of 1:100,000 concentration) over 5–10 minutes followed with IV infusion of 0.1 mcg/kg/min up to 1.5 mcg/kg/min

Asystole: 0.01 mg/kg IV (1:10,000 concentration solution)

Repeat q3–5 min p.r.n.

IV dilution: Dilute 1 mg of 1:1,000 solution with 10 mL 0.9% NS to provide 1:10,000 solution. For infusion, further dilute with 250–500 mL D_5W. For IV infusion, give at 1–10 mcg/min

Nursing Implications

Continuous ECG monitoring is necessary. Excessive doses can cause acute hypertension and arrhythmias.

epoetin alfa (Procrit, Epogen)

Indications

(glycoprotein; erythropoietin)

Used in treatment of anemia in patients receiving chemotherapy, those with chronic renal failure, and HIV-infected patients on zidovudine.

Administration

Given SQ or IV: Initially, 50–100 units/kg administered 1–3 times weekly until desired response

Usual maintenance dosage is 25 units/kg 3 times weekly

IV dilution: No reconstitution is necessary. May be given as an IV bolus

Compatibility: Do not mix with any other medications

Nursing Implications

Avoid excessive agitation of vial; do not shake. Monitor for side effects of fever, hypertension, diarrhea, nausea, or vomiting. Hematocrit and serum iron levels should be monitored frequently.

erythromycin (Many brands)

Indications

(antibiotic; macrolide)

Used in treatment of upper and lower respiratory tract infections, skin infections, pertussis, diphtheria, rheumatic fever, Lyme disease, and chlamydia. Topical preparation used to treat acne. Ophthalmic used to prevent neonatal gonococcal or chlamydial ophthalmia.

Administration

Neonate:

<1.2 kg:	20 mg/kg/24 hr ÷ q12h PO
≥1.2 kg, 0–7 days:	20 mg/kg/24 hr ÷ q12h PO
>7 days:	30 mg/kg/24 hr ÷ q8h PO

Chlamydial conjunctivitis
and pneumonia: 50 mg/kg/24 hr ÷ q6h PO × 14 days

Child: 30–50 mg/kg/24 hr ÷ q6–8h PO (max. dose: 2 g/24 hr)

     20–50 mg/kg/24 hr ÷ q6h IV

Adult: 1–4 g/24 hr ÷ q6h PO (max. dose: 4 g/24 hr)

     15–20 mg/kg/24 hr ÷ q6h IV (max. dose: 4 g/24 hr)

Rheumatic fever prophylaxis: 500 mg/24 hr ÷ q12h PO

Pertussis (Use Estolate salt):   50 mg/kg/24 hr ÷ q6h PO × 14 days

Ophthalmic: Apply 0.5-in. ribbon to affected eye b.i.d.–q.i.d.

IV dilution: Max. concentration: 5 mg/mL

     Usual: 1–2.5 mg/mL over 20–60 min

     Do not give IV push.

Compatibility: D_5W, NS

Nursing Implications

Nausea, vomiting, and abdominal cramps common. Give after meals. Use with caution in liver disease. Can increase digoxin, theophylline, carbamazepine, cyclosporin, and methylprednisolone levels. Ventricular arrhythmias, prolongation of Q-T interval, bradycardia, and hypotension associated with IV use. Prolonging IV infusion duration over ≥60 min has been recommended to decrease cardiotoxic effects.

erythromycin ethylsuccinate and sulfisoxazole acetyl (Pediazole)

Indications

(antibiotic; macrolide and sulfonamide derivative)

Used in treatment of bacterial infections of the upper and lower respiratory tract and OM.

Administration

Child: 50 mg/kg/24 hr erythromycin and 150 mg/kg/24 hr of sulfisoxazole
              ÷ q6h PO *or* 1.25 mL/kg/24 hr ÷ q6h PO (max. dose: 2 g
              erythromycin and 6 g sulfisoxazole/24 hr)

Nursing Implications

Same as erythromycin. Not recommended in infants <2 mo.

fentanyl (Actiq, Duragesic, Fentanyl Transdermal, Sublimaze)

Indications

(narcotic; analgesic; sedative)
    Short-acting analgesic used during anesthesia and in immediate postoperative period. May also be used transdermally to manage chronic pain.

Administration

IV/IM: 1–2 μg/kg/dose q30–60min p.r.n.
Continuous IV: 1 μg/kg/hr; titrate dose to effect; usual range:
                                1–3 μg/kg/hr
IV: For conscious sedation, dose is 0.5–1 μg/kg
Transmucosal lozenge: 10–15 μg/kg for preoperative sedation (not to be
                                used in children <15 kg) 20–40 min before
                                procedure
Transdermal patch: 25 μg/hr for children >12 years and 50 kg
                                Apply to upper torso over dry skin (safety and
                                efficacy have not been established in
                                children <12 yr)
IV dilution: Undiluted slow push over 3–5 min, or if
                                >5 μg/kg over 5–10 min
                                Also can give by continuous infusion

Nursing Implications

Classified as schedule-II drug under FCS Act. Instruct child to suck (not chew) lozenge for 10–20 min. Drug should be used only in monitored setting equipped for emergency airway and ventilation management. Oxygen saturation monitor should be in place. Child should be kept in bed with side rails up during administration. Can cause respiratory depression, apnea, hypotension, bradycardia, and nausea and vomiting.

fluticasone (Flonase, Flovent)

Indications

(corticosteroid; anti-inflammatory)
  Used for relief of seasonal allergic rhinitis. Also used as maintenance treatment of asthma.

Administration

Allergic rhinitis:
  Children > 4 yr: Initially, 100 mcg (1 spray each nostril
                daily) (max. dose: 200 mcg/day)
Asthma:
  Children > 4 yr: 50–100 mcg by inhalation twice daily

Nursing Implications

Frequent side effects include throat irritation, hoarseness, dry mouth, and localized fungal infection in mouth. If patient also uses bronchodilator medications, advise patient to use bronchodilator several minutes before this medication to enhance penetration of steroid into bronchial tree. Teach patient to rinse mouth with water after each inhalation in order to prevent oral fungal infections.

folic acid or folate (Folvite and others)

Indications

(water-soluble vitamin)
  Used to stimulate production of red blood cells, white blood cells, and platelets in anemias caused by folate deficiency. Also reduces risk of neural tube deficits in infants if mother takes before and during pregnancy.

Administration

Folic acid deficiency:

PO/IV/IM/SC	Initial Dose	Maintenance
<1 yr:	15 μg/kg/dose (max. dose: 50 μg/24 hr)	30–45 μg/24 hr
1–10 yr:	1 mg/dose	0.1–0.4 mg/24 hr daily
11 yr–adult:	1–3 mg/dose ÷ daily–t.i.d.	0.5 mg/24 hr daily
Pregnant or lactating:		0.8 mg/24 hr daily
IV dilution:	0.1 mg/mL	

Compatibility: D_5W, NS, SW

Nursing Implications

Urine may appear more yellow. If given IM, give deep IM. Can cause rash, slight flushing, irritability, and GI upset. Normal levels: serum >3 mg/mL.

furosemide (Lasix, Furomide MD, and others)

Indications
(loop diuretic)

Used in management of edema from CHF or hepatic or renal disease and in treatment of hypertension.

Administration

Neonate:	0.5–1 mg/kg/dose q8–24 hr PO/IV/IM (max. dose: 6 mg/kg/dose PO; 2 mg/kg/dose IV)
Infant or child:	0.5–2 mg/kg/dose q6–12 hr PO/IV/IM (max. dose: 6 mg/kg/dose)
Adult:	20–80 mg/24 hr ÷ q6–12h (max. dose: 600 mg/24 hr)
Continuous IV infusion:	
Child or adult:	0.05 mg/kg/hr; titrate to effect
IV dilution:	Undiluted over 1–2 min (max. dose: 0.5 mg/kg/ min (<120 mg)) *or* 4 mg/min (>120 mg)
	Intermittent infusion 1–2 mg/mL (max. dose: 10 mg/mL) over 10–15 min
Compatibility:	D₅W, NS, LR

Nursing Implications
Use cautiously in liver disease. May cause hypokalemia. Observe for dehydration. Oral solutions can cause diarrhea.

gentamicin (Garamycin)

Indications
(antibiotic; aminoglycoside)

Used in treatment of serious gram-negative bacterial infections of the respiratory tract, skin, bone, abdomen, urinary tract, and CNS; endocarditis; and septicemia.

Administration

Neonate:	Doses based on gestational age, postnatal age, and weight. Consult pharmacy or pediatric drug reference.
Child:	6–7.5 mg/kg/24 hr ÷ q8h IV/IM
Adult:	3–6 mg/kg/24 hr ÷ q8h IV/IM
CF:	7.5–10.5 mg/kg/24 hr ÷ q8h IV/IM
IV dilution:	1–2 mg/mL
	Max. concentration: 10 mg/mL over 30–60 min
	Can give by direct injection over 15 min, not to exceed 10 mg/mL
Compatibility:	D₅W, NS, LR

Nursing Implications

Ototoxic and nephrotoxic. Monitor levels. Therapeutic levels: peak: 6–10 mg/L (8–10 in pulmonary infections); trough: <2 mg/L. Administer other IV antibiotics at least 1 hr before or after gentamicin.

glucagon (Glucagon)

Indications

(antihypoglycemic agent)
Used in management of hypoglycemia.

Administration

Neonate or infant:	0.025–0.3 mg/kg/dose q30min p.r.n. IV/IM/SC (max. dose: 1 mg/dose)
Child:	0.03–0.1 mg/kg/dose q20min p.r.n. IV/IM/SC (max. dose: 1 mg/dose)
Adult:	0.5–1 mg/dose q20min p.r.n. IV/IM/SC
IV dilution:	
Direct IV:	Dilute with manufacturer's diluent, resulting in 1-mg/mL concentration
	If doses >2 mg are used, dilute with SW instead of diluent
Compatibility:	All dextrose solutions; will precipitate with NS

Nursing Implications

High doses have cardiac stimulatory effect and have been used in β-blocker overdoses. Can cause nausea, vomiting, urticaria, and respiratory distress.

griseofulvin (Grifulvin V, Grisactin, Fulvicin, Gris-PEG)

Indications

(antifungal agent)
Used in treatment of tinea infections of the skin, hair, and nails.

Administration

Microsize:	
Child:	10–20 mg/kg/24 hr ÷ daily–b.i.d. PO
Adult:	500–1,000 mg/24 hr ÷ daily–b.i.d. PO (max. dose: 1 g/ 24 hr)
Ultramicrosize:	
Child >2 yr:	5–10 mg/kg/24 hr ÷ daily–b.i.d. PO
Adult:	330–750 mg/24 hr ÷ daily–b.i.d. PO (max. dose: 750 mg/ 24 hr)

Nursing Implications

Give with milk, eggs, or fatty foods to increase absorption. Usual treatment period 4–6 wk for tinea capitis, 4–6 mo for tinea unguium. May cause leukopenia. Monitor hematologic, renal, and hepatic function, especially for courses >4–6 wk. May decrease effectiveness of oral contraceptive pills (OCPs).

haloperidol (Haldol)
Indications

(antipsychotic; antiemetic, antidyskinetic)

Used for treatment of psychoses, Tourette's disorder, severe behavioral problems in children, and emergency sedation of acutely agitated patients.

Administration

3–12 yr (15–40 kg):	Initially, 0.25–0.5 mg/day PO in divided doses (max. dosage not to exceed 0.15 mg/kg/day)
6–12 yr:	1–3 mg/dose IM q4–8h (max. dosage not to exceed 0.15 mg/kg/day)

Nursing Implications

Monitor for side effects of blurred vision, constipation, dry mouth, and hypotension. After IM administration, patient must remain recumbent for 30–60 minutes in head-low position with legs raised to minimize hypotension.

hydromorphone (Dilaudid)
Indications

(opioid agonist; narcotic analgesic; antitussive)

Relief of moderate to severe pain, persistent nonproductive cough.

Administration

Analgesia:

Children > 12 yr:	1–4 mg/dose PO/SQ/IM/IV q4–6h
Children < 12 yr:	0.015 mg/kg/dose IV q4–6h
	0.03–0.08 mg/kg/dose PO q4–6h (max. 5 mg)

Antitussive:

Children >12 yr:	1 mg q3–4h
Children 6–12 yr:	0.5 mg q3–4h
IV dilution:	May give undiluted. Administer IV push very slowly (over 2–5 min)
Compatibility:	0.9% NaCl

Nursing Implications

Side effects depend upon dosage and route of administration. Patients may complain of dizziness, nausea, and vomiting. Advise patient to increase fiber, fluids, and exercise to prevent constipation. Monitor patient for any signs of respiratory depression and hypotension.

hydroxyzine (Atarax, Vistaril)

Indications

(antihistamine; anxiolytic)

Used in treatment of anxiety, for preoperative sedation, and as an antiemetic and antipruritic.

Administration

Child: 2 mg/kg/24 hr ÷ q6–8h PO
         0.5–1 mg/kg/dose q4–6h p.r.n. IM
Adult: 25–100 mg/dose q4–6h p.r.n. PO/IM (max. dose: 600 mg/24 hr)

Nursing Implications

Potentiates barbiturates, meperidine, and other depressants. Can cause dry mouth, drowsiness, tremor, convulsions, blurred vision, and hypotension. IV not recommended but has been administered by slow IV to oncology patients via CVLs without problems.

ibuprofen (Motrin, Advil, and others)

Indications

(NSAID)

Used in management of inflammatory disorders such as juvenile rheumatoid arthritis (JRA) and as analgesic for mild to moderate pain. Also used for dysmenorrhea, gout, and fever.

Administration

Child:

Analgesic or antipyretic:	5–10 mg/kg/dose q6–8h PO (max. dose: 40 mg/kg/24 hr PO)
JRA:	30–50 mg/kg/24 hr ÷ q6h PO (max. dose: 2,400 mg/24 hr PO)

Adult:

Inflammatory disease:	400–800 mg/dose q6–8h PO
Pain, fever, or dysmenorrhea:	200–400 mg/dose q4–6h PO (max. dose: 3.2 g/24 hr PO)

Nursing Implications

Use with caution in liver and renal impairment. Can cause nausea, vomiting, rash, and ocular problems. Also can cause granulocytopenia and anemia and inhibit platelet aggregation. May increase serum levels and effects of digoxin, methotrexate, and lithium. May decrease effects of antihypertensives, furosemide, and thiazide diuretics. GI problems can be lessened by administering with milk.

imipramine (Tofranil, Janimine)

Indications

(antidepressant, tricyclic)

Used to treat various forms of depression, enuresis in children, and as analgesic for certain chronic and neuropathic pain.

Administration

Antidepressant:

Child:	Initial: 1.5 mg/kg/24 hr ÷ t.i.d. PO; increase 1–1.5 mg/kg/24 hr q3–4days (max. dose: 5 mg/kg/24 hr)
Adolescent:	Initial: 25–50 mg/24 hr ÷ daily–t.i.d. PO; doses >100 mg/24 hr usually not needed
Adult:	Initial: 75–100 mg/24 hr ÷ t.i.d. PO/IM (max. dose: 100 mg/24 hr) Maintenance: 50–300 mg/24 hr q.h.s. PO (max. PO dose: 300 mg/24 hr)
Enuresis (≥6 yr):	Initial: 10–25 mg q.h.s. Increment: 10–25 mg/dose at 1- to 2-wk intervals until max. dose for age or desired effect achieved Continue for 2–3 mo, then taper slowly. (max. dose: 6–12 yr: 50 mg/24 hr; 12–14 yr: 75 mg/24 hr)
Chronic pain:	Initial: 0.2–0.4 mg/kg/dose q.h.s. PO; increase 50% q2–3days (max. dose: 1–3 mg/kg/dose q.h.s. PO)

Nursing Implications

Can cause hypotension, sedation, urinary retention, constipation, dry mouth, dizziness, drowsiness, and arrhythmia. PO route preferred. *Do not discontinue abruptly in patients receiving long-term high-dose therapy.*

ipratropium bromide (Atrovent)

Indications

(anticholinergic agent)

Bronchodilator used in treatment of bronchospasm associated with asthma, chronic obstructive pulmonary disease (COPD), bronchitis, and emphysema. Also used for symptomatic relief of rhinorrhea associated with allergic and nonallergic rhinitis.

Administration
Inhaler:
<12 yr:	1–2 puffs t.i.d.–q.i.d.
≥12 yr:	2–3 puffs q.i.d. up to 12 puffs/24 hr

Nebulized:
Neonate:	25 μg/kg/dose t.i.d.
Infant or child:	250 μg/dose t.i.d.–q.i.d.
>12 yr–adult:	250–500 μg/dose t.i.d.–q.i.d.

Nasal spray:
>12 yr–adult:	2 sprays per nostril b.i.d.–t.i.d.

Nursing Implications
Use with caution in patients with narrow angle glaucoma and bladder neck obstruction. May cause anxiety, dizziness, HA, GI discomfort, and cough with inhaled and nebulized doses. Nasal spray can cause nasal congestion and dry mouth. Shake inhaler well before use. Use spacer in children <8 yr. Nebulized solution can be mixed with albuterol.

iron (Fe) (Fer-In-Sol and others)
Indications
(oral iron supplements)
Used in prevention and treatment of iron-deficiency anemias.

Administration
Treatment:
Preterm:	2–4 mg elemental Fe/kg/24 hr ÷ daily–b.i.d. PO (max. dose: 15 mg elemental Fe/24 hr)
Child:	3–6 mg elemental Fe/kg/24 hr ÷ daily–t.i.d. PO
Adult:	60 mg elemental Fe b.i.d.–q.i.d.

Prevention:
Preterm:	2 mg elemental Fe/kg/24 hr
Term or child:	1–2 mg elemental Fe/kg/24 hr (max. dose: 15 mg elemental Fe/24 hr)
Adult:	60–100 mg elemental Fe/24 hr PO ÷ daily–b.i.d.

Nursing Implications
Liquid preparations stain teeth. Use dropper or straw to administer. Less GI irritation if given with or after meals. Do not give with milk or milk products. May cause constipation, dark stools, nausea, and epigastric pain.

kanamycin (Kantrex)

Indications

(antibiotic; aminoglycoside)

Used in treatment of gram-negative bacillary and staphylococcal infections of bone, respiratory tract, skin, and abdomen; complicated UTIs; endocarditis; and septicemia.

Administration

Neonate:

<7 days, <2 kg:	15 mg/kg/24 hr ÷ q12h IV/IM
≥2 kg:	20 mg/kg/24 hr ÷ q12h IV/IM
≥7 days, <2 kg:	22.5 mg/kg/24 hr ÷ q8h IV/IM
≥2 kg:	30 mg/kg/24 hr ÷ q8h IV/IM
Infant or child:	15–30 mg/kg/24 hr ÷ q8–12h IV/IM
Adult:	15 mg/kg/24 hr ÷ q8–12h IV/IM
PO for GI bacterial overgrowth:	150–250 mg/kg/24 hr ÷ q6h (max. dose: 4 g/24 hr)
IV dilution:	2.5–5 mg/mL over 30–60 min
	Do not give IV push.
	37.5 mg/mL via CVL
Compatibility:	D_5W, NS, LR, $D_{10}W$

Nursing Implications

Renal toxicity and ototoxicity may occur. Poorly absorbed orally, so only used PO to treat GI bacterial overgrowth. Therapeutic levels: peak: 15–30 mg/L; trough: <5–10 mg/L.

ketoconazole (Nizoral)

Indications

(antifungal agent)

Used to treat topical and systemic fungal infections and as suppressive therapy against mucocutaneous candidiasis in HIV patients.

Administration

Oral:

Child ≥2 yr:	3.3–6.6 mg/kg/24 hr daily
Adult:	200–400 mg/24 hr daily (max. dose: 800 mg/24 hr ÷ b.i.d.)
Topical:	1–2 applications/24 hr
Shampoo:	Twice weekly × 4 wk with at least 3 days between applications, and intermittently as needed to maintain control

Suppressive treatment:
    Child: 5–10 mg/kg/24 hr ÷ daily–b.i.d. PO
    Adolescent or adult: 200 mg/dose daily PO

Nursing Implications

Monitor LFTs in long-term use. May cause nausea, vomiting, rash, HA, pruritus, and fever. Contraindicated in patients on terfenadine because of possible cardiac arrhythmias. May increase effects and levels of phenytoin, digoxin, cyclosporin, protease inhibitors, and warfarin. Phenobarbital, rifampin, INH, H_2-blockers, antacids, and omeprazole can decrease levels of ketoconazole.

loratidine (Claritin)
Indications

(antihistamine)
    Used to treat symptoms of seasonal allergic rhinitis (hayfever) and urticaria.

Administration

Children >6 yr: 10 mg PO once daily
Children 2–5 yr: 5 mg PO once daily

Nursing Implications

Side effects include headache, fatigue, and drowsiness. Advise patient to drink adequate amount of water to prevent dry mouth.

lorazepam (Ativan)
Indications

(benzodiazepine anticonvulsant)
    Used in management of anxiety and status epilepticus and for preoperative sedation and amnesia. Also used for antiemetic adjunct therapy.

Administration

Status epilepticus:
    Neonate, infant,   0.05–0.1 mg/kg/dose over 2–5 min IV; may repeat
      child, or adolescent: 0.05 mg × 1 in 10–15 min (max. dose: 4 mg/
                      dose)
    Adult: 4 mg/dose slowly over 2–5 min IV; may repeat in
                      5–15 min (total max. dose in 12-hr period is
                      8 mg)
Antiemetic adjunct:
    Child: 0.04–0.08 mg/kg/dose q6h p.r.n. IV (max. single
                      dose: 4 mg)

Anxiolytic or sedation:

Child:	0.05 mg/kg/dose q4–8h IV/PO *or* IM for procedural sedation (max. dose: 2 mg/dose)
Adult:	1–10 mg/24 hr ÷ b.i.d.–t.i.d. PO
IV dilution:	Do not exceed 2 mg/min or 0.05 mg/kg over 2–5 min
Compatibility:	D_5W, NS, SW

Nursing Implications

Injectable form contains 2% benzyl alcohol, which may be toxic to neonates in high doses. Aspirate repeatedly when giving IV to make sure injection is not intraarterial and that perivascular extravasation has not occurred. Injectable form may also be given rectally. May cause respiratory depression, sedation, dizziness, mild ataxia, mood changes, rash, and GI symptoms.

mannitol (Osmitrol, Resectisol)

Indications

(osmotic diuretic)

Used to reduce increased intracranial pressure (ICP) associated with cerebral edema, to promote diuresis in prevention or treatment of oliguria or anuria resulting from acute renal failure, to reduce increased ocular pressure, and to promote urinary excretion of toxic substances.

Administration

Anuria or oliguria:

Test dose (to assess renal function):	0.2 g/kg/dose IV (max. dose: 12.5 g over 3–5 min) If no diuresis, mannitol is discontinued.
Initial:	0.5–1 g/kg/dose IV
Maintenance:	0.25–0.5 g/kg/dose q4–6h IV
Cerebral edema:	0.25 g/kg/dose IV over 20–30 min; gradually increased to 1 g/kg/dose if needed
IV administration:	In-line filter set (≤5 micron) should always be used for infusion with concentrations ≥20%; test dose given IV push over 3–5 min; for cerebral edema or elevated ICP, administer over 20–30 min

Compatibility: Do not mix with IV fluids. NaCl and KCl can cause precipitation.

Nursing Implications

Do not use solutions that contain crystals. Hot water bath and vigorous shaking may be used to dissolve crystals. Contraindicated in severe renal disease, active intracranial bleed, dehydration, and pulmonary edema. May cause circulatory overload, electrolyte disturbances, hypovolemia, HA, and polydipsia.

meperidine hydrochloride (Demerol and others)

Indications

(narcotic; analgesic)

Used in management of moderate to severe pain. Also used for preoperative sedation.

Administration

PO, IV, IM, or SC:

Child:	1–1.5 mg/kg/dose q3–4h p.r.n. (max. dose: 100 mg)
Adult:	50–150 mg/dose q3–4h p.r.n.
IV dilution:	≤10 mg/mL direct IV slowly over ≥5 min
Intermittent infusion:	1 mg/mL over 15–30 min
Infusion:	0.3–0.7 mg/kg/hr
Compatibility:	D₅W, NS, LR, D₁₀W

Nursing Implication

IV dose lower. Contraindicated in patients with cardiac arrhythmias, asthma, and increased ICP. Can cause nausea, vomiting, respiratory depression, smooth muscle spasm, pruritus, palpitations, hypotension, constipation, and lethargy. Continued use decreases effects. Not recommended for chronic use. Dilute PO syrup in water before use.

meropenem (Merrem)

Indications

(antibiotic)

Used in treatment of multidrug-resistant gram-negative and gram-positive aerobic and anaerobic pathogens and for treatment of meningitis; lower respiratory tract, urinary tract, intraabdominal, and skin infections; and sepsis.

Administration

Child ≥3 mo:	60 mg/kg/24 hr ÷ q8h IV
Meningitis:	120 mg/kg/24 hr ÷ q8h IV (max. dose: 6 g/24 hr)

Adult:
Mild-to-moderate
infection: 1.5–3 g/24 hr ÷ q8h IV
Meningitis: 6 g/24 hr ÷ q8h IV
IV dilution:
Direct IV: Max. concentration: 50 mg/mL over 3–5 min
Intermittent infusion: 50 mg/mL over 15–30 min
Compatibility: D_5W, NS, SW

Nursing Implications

Probenecid inhibits renal excretion. Safety not established for children
<3 mo. Use with caution in patients with history of seizures, with CNS
disease or infection, or with decreased renal function. Can cause pseudomembranous colitis; hypotension; rash; nausea and vomiting; diarrhea;
neutropenia; increased LFTs, BUN, and creatinine; and dyspnea. Prolonged
use may result in superinfection.

metaproterenol (Alupent)

Indications

(bronchodilator)
Used to treat reversible bronchospasm due to bronchial asthma and bronchitis.

Administration

Children > 9 yr: 20 mg PO 3–4 times/day
                    2–3 inhalations q3–4h (maximum of 12 inhalations/24 hrs)
                    10–15 mg (0.2–0.3 mL) of 5% solution via nebulizer
Children 6–9 yr: 10 mg PO 3–4 times/day
                    0.5–1 mg/kg (0.01–0.02 mL/kg) of 5% solution via
                      nebulizer
Children 2–6 yr: 1.3–2.6 mg/kg/day PO in 3–4 divided doses
                    0.5–1 mg/kg (0.01–0.02 mL/kg) of 5% solution via
                      nebulizer
Children < 2 yr: 0.4 mg/kg PO 3–4 times daily
                    0.5–1 mg/kg (0.01–0.02 mL/kg) of 5% solution via
                      nebulizer

Nursing Implications

Monitor for therapeutic effect of relieving bronchospasm. Side effects
include palpitations, nervousness, restlessness, tachycardia, chills, and
sweating.

methicillin (Staphcillin)
Indications
(antibiotic; penicillin, penicillinase-resistant)

Used in treatment of respiratory tract, skin, bone, joint, and urinary tract infections; and endocarditis, septicemia, and CNS infections caused by susceptible strains of penicillinase-producing *Staphylococcus*.

Administration
Neonate:

≤7 days, <2 kg:	50–100 mg/kg/24 hr ÷ q12h IV/IM
≥2 kg:	75–150 mg/kg/24 hr ÷ q8h IV/IM
>7 days, <1.2 kg:	50–100 mg/kg/24 hr ÷ q12h IV/IM
1.2–2 kg:	75–150 mg/kg/24 hr ÷ q8h IV/IM
≥2 kg:	100–200 mg/kg/24 hr ÷ q8h IV/IM
Infant >1 mo/child:	150–400 mg/kg/24 hr ÷ q4–6h IV/IM
Adult:	4–12 g/24 hr ÷ q4–6h IV/IM (max. dose: 12 g/24 hr)
IV dilution:	2–20 mg/mL over 15–30 min
Compatibility:	D5W, NS, LR

Nursing Implications
Administer IM dose deep in large muscle mass using solution with concentration of 500 mg/mL. May cause hematuria, reversible bone marrow depression, hairy tongue, positive Coombs' test and rash, and phlebitis at IV site. Has been associated with interstitial nephritis and hemorrhagic cystitis.

methylphenidate (Ritalin)
Indications
(CNS stimulant)

Used to treat children with ADHD and narcolepsy.

Administration

Initial:	0.3 mg/kg/dose (*or* 2.5–5 mg/dose) given before breakfast and lunch. May increase by 0.1 mg/kg/dose (*or* 5–10 mg/ 24 hr) weekly until maintenance dose achieved. May need to give extra afternoon dose.
Maintenance:	0.3–1 mg/kg/24 hr (max. dose: 2 mg/kg/24 hr *or* 60 mg/24 hr)

Nursing Implications
Classified as schedule-II drug under FCS Act. Avoid administration in evening so sleep is not interrupted; however, children with severe ADHD may need dose to calm them enough to go to sleep. Assess child's behavior

through caregiver and teacher report in regard to concentration ability. Client should be taught to take drug as prescribed. Tapering may be needed when drug is being discontinued. Safe storage is an issue because this drug has potential for street abuse. Should be transported to school by an adult. Child should be observed swallowing pill. High dose may slow growth through appetite suppression. Dose may need to be given after meals for children with appetite suppression. Contraindicated in clients with glaucoma, anxiety disorders, motor tics, and Tourette's syndrome. Can cause insomnia, weight loss, anorexia, rash, nausea, vomiting, abdominal pain, hypertension or hypotension, tachycardia, arrhythmias, palpitations, restlessness, HA, fever, tremor, and thrombocytopenia.

methylprednisolone (Medrol, Solu-Medrol, and others)

Indications

(corticosteroid)

Used in management of chronic inflammatory, allergic, hematologic, neoplastic, and autoimmune diseases.

Administration

Anti-inflammatory or immunosuppressive:	0.5–1.7 mg/kg/24 hr ÷ q6–12h PO/IV/IM
Status asthmaticus:	
Child:	
Loading:	2 mg/kg/dose IV/IM × 1
Maintenance:	2 mg/kg/24 hr ÷ q6h IV/IM
Adult:	10–250 mg/dose q4–6h IV/IM
IV dilution:	Undiluted for push (max. concentration: 62.5 mg/ mL over 3–5 min)
	Do not administer high dose (15 mg/kg or ≥500 mg/dose) *by IV push.*
Infusion:	2.5–5 mg/mL over 15–60 min
Compatibility:	D_5W, NS

Nursing Implications

Monitor BP with IV infusion. Hypotension, cardiac arrhythmia, and sudden death have been reported in patients given high-dose methylprednisolone IV push over <20 min. Do not give acetate form IV. Can cause same type of side effects with long-term use as other corticosteroids. Should never be discontinued abruptly.

metoclopramide (Reglan, Clopra, Maxolon, and others)

Indications

(antiemetic; prokinetic agent)

Used in treatment of GE reflux and in prevention and treatment of nausea and vomiting associated with chemotherapy and postoperatively.

Administration

GE reflux:

Infant or child:	0.1–0.2 mg/kg/dose up to q.i.d. IV/IM/PO (max. dose: 0.8 mg/kg/24 hr)
Adult:	10–15 mg/dose a.c. and q. h.s. IV/IM/PO
Antiemetic:	1–2 mg/kg/dose q2–6h IV/IM/PO
IV dilution:	0.2 mg/mL max. concentration: 5 mg/mL over 15–30 min (max. rate 5 mg/min)
Compatibility:	D$_5$W, NS, LR

Nursing Implications

Contraindicated in GI obstruction, seizure disorder, and pheochromocytoma or in patients receiving drugs likely to cause extrapyramidal symptoms (EPS). May cause EPS, sedation, HA, anxiety, leukopenia, and diarrhea. Give PO dose 30 min a.c. and h.s. for GE reflux.

metronidazole (Flagyl)

Indications

(antibacterial; antiprotozoal)

Used to treat anaerobic infections (skin, CNS, lower respiratory tract, bone and joints, intra-abdominal, gynecological, septicemia).

Administration

Anaerobic bacterial infections:

30 mg/kg/day IV/PO in 4 divided doses (not to exceed 4 g/day)

Treatment usually begins with IV route, then orally

Amebiasis:

35–50 mg/kg/day PO in 3 divided doses

Other parasitic infections:

15–30 mg/kg/day PO in 3 divided doses

IV dilution:	Comes prepared in ready-to-use infusion bag. Infuse over 60 min Do not give as a bolus

Nursing Implications

Oral doses may be taken with food to minimize GI upset. Urine color may change to reddish-brown or dark while taking this medication.

midazolam (Versed)

Indications

(benzodiazepine)

Used for sedation, anxiolysis, and amnesia before a procedure or anesthesia; conscious sedation for procedures; and continuous sedation of intubated and mechanically ventilated patients. Also sometimes used in status epilepticus.

Administration

Doses titrated to effect under controlled conditions.
Procedural sedation:
PO:
Infant ≥6 mo/child: Single dose, 0.25–0.5 mg/kg/dose; usual dose, 0.5 mg/kg (max. dose: 20 mg)
IM:
Child: Usual dose, 0.1–0.15 mg/kg/dose 30–60 min before procedure or surgery (max. total dose: 10 mg)
IV:
6 mo–5 yr: 0.05–0.1 mg/kg/dose over 2–3 min; may repeat p.r.n. q2–3min (max. total dose: 6 mg)
6–12 yr: 0.025–0.05 mg/kg/dose over 2–3 min; may repeat p.r.n. q2–3min (max. total dose: 10 mg)
>12–16 yr: Use adult dose up to max. total dose of 10 mg
Adult: 0.5–2 mg/dose over 2 min; may repeat p.r.n. q2–3min (Usual total dose: 2.5–5 mg)
Sedation with mechanical ventilation:
Intermittent IV:
Infant or child: 0.05–0.15 mg/kg/dose q1–2h p.r.n.
Continuous IV infusion:
Neonate:
<32 wk gestation: 0.5 μg/kg/min
≥32 wk gestation: 1 μg/kg/min
Infant or child: 1–2 μg/kg/min

IV dilution: 1–5 mg/mL over ≥2–5 min *or* by infusion as above

Compatibility: D_5W or 0.9% NaCl

Nursing Implications

Do not give intraarterially. Give PO on empty stomach. Cardiovascular monitoring recommended. Can cause respiratory depression, hypotension, and bradycardia.

montelukast (Singulair)

Indications

(antiasthmatic; leukotriene receptor antagonist)
    Used for prophylaxis and chronic treatment of asthma.

Administration

Child 6–14 yr: Chew 5-mg chewable tablet q. h.s. PO
>15 yr–adult: 10 mg q. h.s. PO

Nursing Implications

Contraindicated in phenylketonuric patients. Phenobarbital and rifampin increase clearance of montelukast. Possible side effects include HA, nausea, abdominal pain, diarrhea, dyspepsia, fatigue, dizziness, elevated liver enzymes, cough, laryngitis, pharyngitis, otitis, sinusitis, and viral infections.

morphine sulfate (Many brands)

Indications

(narcotic; analgesic)
    Used in management of severe acute and chronic pain. Effective with painful sickle cell crisis and cyanotic spells associated with tetralogy.

Administration

Doses titrated to effect.
Analgesia or tetralogy
    spells:
        Neonate: 0.05–0.2 mg/kg/dose q4h slow IV/IM/SC
        Neonate opiate
            withdrawal: 0.08–0.2 mg/dose q3–4h slow IV/IM/SC
        Infant or child: 0.2–0.5 mg/kg/dose q4–6h p.r.n. PO (immediate release)
                          0.3–0.6 mg/kg/dose q12h PO (controlled release)
                          0.1–0.2 mg/kg/dose q2–4h p.r.n. IV/IM/SC (max. dose: 15 mg/dose)

Adult:	10–30 mg q4h p.r.n. PO (immediate release)
	15–30 mg q8–12h p.r.n. PO (controlled release)
	2–15 mg/dose q2–6h p.r.n. IV/IM/SC

Continuous IV:
Neonate:	0.01–0.02 mg/kg/hr
Infant or child:	0.025–2.6 mg/kg/hr
Adult:	0.8–10 mg/hr

IV dilution:
Direct IV:	0.5–5 mg/mL over 5 min
Intermittent IV:	over 15–30 min
Continuous IV:	0.1–1 mg/mL
Compatibility:	D_5W

Nursing Implications

Give PO dose with food. Rapid IV administration may increase adverse effects. Can cause dependence, CNS and respiratory depression, nausea, vomiting, urinary retention, hypotension, constipation, bradycardia, and increased ICP. Causes histamine release resulting in itching and possible bronchospasm. Assess for sedation and respiratory depression. Naloxone may be used to reverse effects.

nafcillin (Unipen, Nafcil, and others)

Indications

(antibiotic; penicillin, penicillinase resistant)

Used in treatment of penicillinase-producing staphylococci infections of respiratory tract, bone, joints, skin, and urinary tract. Also used in endocarditis, septicemia, and CNS infections.

Administration

Neonate:	
≤7 days, <2 kg:	50 mg/kg/24 hr ÷ q12h IV/IM
≥2 kg:	75 mg/kg/24 hr ÷ q8h IV/IM
>7 days, <1.2 kg:	50 mg/kg/24 hr ÷ q12h IV/IM
1.2–2 kg:	75 mg/kg/24 hr ÷ q8h IV/IM
≥2 kg:	100 mg/kg/24 hr ÷ q6h IV/IM
>7 days:	75 mg/kg/24 hr ÷ q6h IV/IM
Infant or child:	50–100 mg/kg/24 hr ÷ q6h PO
Mild to moderate infections:	50–100 mg/kg/24 hr ÷ q6h IV/IM
Severe infections:	100–200 mg/kg/24 hr ÷ q4–6h IV/IM
Adult:	250–1,000 mg q4–6h PO
	500–2,000 mg q4–6h IV
	500 mg q4–6h IM (max. dose: 12 g/24 hr)

IV dilution:	10–40 mg/mL over 60 min
Compatibility:	D$_5$W, NS, LR, D$_{10}$W

Nursing Implications

Give PO on empty stomach. Give IM deep into large muscle at 250 mg/mL. High incidence of phlebitis with IV route that can cause tissue sloughing and necrosis. Decrease rate or concentration for vein irritation. Sodium bicarbonate may be added to IV dilution to buffer effects. Warm or cold compresses at IV site may help decrease pain during infusion.

naloxone (Narcan)
Indications

(narcotic antagonist; antidote)

Used to treat opioid toxicity and opioid-induced respiratory depression.

Administration

Opioid toxicity:	0.1 mg/kg IV/IM/SQ (IV preferred) to a dose of 2 mg administered q2–3min until 5 doses (up to 10 mg) have been given
Opioid respiratory depression:	5–10 mcg (0.005–0.01 mg) q2–3min
IV dilution:	Dilute 1 mg/mL with 50 mL Sterile Water for Injection to provide a concentration of 0.02 mg/mL
	For continuous IV infusion, dilute 2 mg of naloxone with 500 mg of D$_5$W or 0.9% NaCl, producing a solution containing 0.004 mg/mL
Compatibility	D$_5$W, 0.9% NaCl

Nursing Implications

Too rapid reversal of narcotic depression can result in vomiting, nausea, sweating, increased BP, and tachycardia. Observe patient after satisfactory response because duration of opiate may exceed duration of Narcan, resulting in recurrence of respiratory depression.

naproxen/naproxen sodium (Naprosyn, Anaprox, Aleve [over the counter])
Indications

(NSAID)

Used to manage inflammatory disease and rheumatoid disorders including JRA; acute gout, mild to moderate pain; and dysmenorrhea.

Administration

All doses based on naproxen base.

Child >2 yr:

Analgesia:	5–7 mg/kg/dose q8–12h PO
JRA:	10–20 mg/kg/24 hr ÷ q12h PO (max. dose: 1,250 mg/24 hr)

Rheumatoid arthritis or
  ankylosing spondylitis:

Adult:	250–500 mg b.i.d. PO
Dysmenorrhea:	500 mg × 1, then 250 mg q6–8h PO (max. dose: 1,250 mg/24 hr)

Nursing Implications

May cause GI bleeding, thrombocytopenia, heartburn, HA, drowsiness, vertigo, and tinnitus. Use with caution in patients with GI disease, cardiac disease, or renal or hepatic impairment, and in those on anticoagulants. Give with food to decrease GI effects.

nitrofurantoin (Furadantin, Macrodantin)

Indications

(antibiotic)
  Used for prevention and treatment of UTIs.

Administration

Child >1 mo:

Treatment:	5–7 mg/kg/24h ÷ q6h PO (max. dose: 400 mg/24 hr)
Prophylaxis:	1–2 mg/kg/dose q. h.s. PO (max. dose: 100 mg/24 hr)

Adult:

Treatment:	50–100 mg/dose q6h PO (for dual release: 100 mg/dose q12h PO)
Prophylaxis:	50–100 mg PO q. h.s.

Nursing Implications

Can cause nausea, vomiting, HA, and false-positive urine glucose. Contraindicated in severe renal disease and G6PD deficiency, and in infants <1 mo. Give with food or milk.

nystatin (Mycostatin, Nilstat, and others)

Indications

(antifungal agent)
  PO, topical, and vaginal treatment of candidal infections.

Administration

Oral:

Preterm infant:	0.5 mL (50,000 units) to each side of mouth q.i.d.
Term infant:	1 mL (100,000 units) to each side of mouth q.i.d.
Child or adult:	
Suspension:	4–6 mL (400,000–600,000 units) swish and swallow q.i.d.
Troche:	200,000–400,000 units 4–5x/24 hr
Vaginal:	1 tablet q. h.s. × 10 days
Topical:	Apply to affected area b.i.d.–q.i.d.

Nursing Implications

May need to paint on lesions in mouth with cotton swab or clean pacifier with infants. Nipples and pacifiers need to be cleaned thoroughly. Troches must be allowed to dissolve slowly and must not be chewed or swallowed whole. Can cause GI effects. Must continue to treat until 48–72 hr after lesions are gone. For mothers with candidal infection of skin around areola who are breastfeeding their infants, suspension can be rubbed on breasts.

omeprazole (Prilosec)

Indications

(gastic acid pump inhibitor)

Used for short-term treatment of erosive esophagitis, symptomatic gastroesophageal reflux disease (GERD).

Administration

2 yr and older (< 20 kg):
      10 mg/day PO
2 yr and older (> 20 kg):
      20 mg/day PO

Nursing Implications

Give before meals making sure not to crush or chew capsules. Side effects of headache, diarrhea, and abdominal pain should be monitored.

oseltamivir (Tamiflu)

Indications

(antiviral)

Used for symptomatic treatment of uncomplicated acute illness caused by influenza A or B virus in children over age 1 who are symptomatic no longer than 2 days. Also used to prevent influenza in children >13 years.

Administration

Children < 15 kg: 30 mg PO b.i.d.
Children 15–23 kg: 45 mg PO b.i.d.
Children 23–40 kg: 60 mg PO b.i.d.
Children > 40 kg: 75 mg PO b.i.d.

Nursing Implications

Nausea, vomiting, and diarrhea are the most frequent side effects. To have maximum effectiveness, drug therapy should be started at first appearance of flu symptoms. Counsel patients that this is not a substitute for the flu shot.

palivizumab (Synagis)

Indications

(monoclonal antibody)

Used to prevent serious disease caused by respiratory syncytial virus (RSV) in infants with chronic lung disease <2 yr old and infants who were born at <35 weeks' gestation and are <12 mo old. Given during RSV season, typically November through April.

Administration

15 mg/kg/dose IM q mo during RSV season

Nursing Implications

IM is only current route. Administer in anterolateral aspect of thigh. Reconstitute with 1 mL SW for injection and gently swirl to mix. Dose should be given within 6 hr of mixing. Volumes >1 mL should be given as divided dose. May see slight increase in incidence of rhinitis, rash, pain, increased LFTs, pharyngitis, cough, wheeze, diarrhea, vomiting, conjunctivitis, and anemia.

pemoline (Cylert)

Indications

(CNS stimulant)

Used in children for treatment of ADHD and narcolepsy.

Administration

Child ≥6 yr:
    Initial: 37.5 mg q AM PO; increase in 18.75-mg/24 hr
                           increments q wk
    Maintenance: 0.5–3 mg/kg/24 hr (effective range: 56.25–75 mg/24 hr)
                           (max. dose: 112.5 mg/24 hr)

Nursing Implications

Classified as schedule-IV drug by FCS Act. Liver enzyme studies recommended before therapy; if elevated, drug should not be used. Baseline growth indices are plotted on growth grids and monitored while child is taking medication. Obtain periodic reports from caregivers and teachers regarding behavior. May take 3–4 wk for positive changes in child's behavior. Drug can produce dependence and abuse is a potential. May cause insomnia, HA, seizures, anorexia, depression, abdominal pain, movement disorders, and hepatotoxicity. Contraindicated in patients with Tourette's syndrome.

penicillin G (benzathine preparations) (Bicillin L-A)

Indications

(antibiotic; penicillin, very long-acting IM)

Used in treatment of mild to moderate infections, such as group A streptococcal pharyngitis, and to prevent rheumatic fever.

Administration

Group A streptococci:

Infant or child:	25,000–50,000 units/kg/dose × 1 IM
	Max. dose: 1.2 million units/dose *or*
>1 mo, <27 kg:	600,000 units/dose × 1 IM
≥27 kg–adult:	1.2 million units/dose × 1 IM

Rheumatic fever prophylaxis:

Infant or child:	25,000–50,000 units/kg IM q3–4 wk (max. dose: 1.2 million units/dose)
Adult:	1.2 million units/dose IM q3–4 wk *or* 600,000 units/dose IM q2wk
Compatibility:	Sterile H_2O for injection

Nursing Implications

Do not give IV. Side effects similar to those in aqueous penicillin G. Provides sustained levels for 2–4 wk. Not recommended for treatment of congenital syphilis.

penicillin G (potassium and sodium preparations) (Many brands)

Indications

(antibiotic; aqueous penicillin)

Used in treatment of pneumonia, sepsis, group B streptococcal meningitis, syphilis, and gonorrhea.

Administration

Neonate:

≤7 days, ≤2 kg:	50,000–100,000 units/kg/24 hr ÷ q12h IV/IM
>2 kg:	75,000–150,000 units/kg/24 hr ÷ q8h IV/IM
>7 days, <1.2 kg:	50,000–100,000 units/kg/24 hr ÷ q12h IV/IM
1.2–2 kg:	75,000–150,000 units/kg/24 hr ÷ q8h IV/IM
≥2 kg:	100,000–200,000 units/kg/24 hr ÷ q6h IV/IM

Congenital syphilis:

≤7 days:	100,000 units/kg/24 hr ÷ q12h IV/IM
>7 days:	150,000 units/kg/24 hr ÷ q8h IV/IM

Group B streptococcal meningitis:

≤7 days:	250,000–450,000 units/kg/24 hr ÷ q8h IV/IM
>7 days:	450,000 units/kg/24 hr ÷ q6h IV/IM
Infant or child:	100,000–400,000 units/kg/24 hr ÷ q4–6h IV/IM (max. dose: 24 million units/24 hr)
Adult:	4–24 million units/24 hr ÷ q4–6h IV/IM
IV dilution:	100,000–500,000 units/mL over 15–60 min
	50,000 units/mL over 15–30 min recommended for neonates or infants
Compatibility:	D_5W, NS, LR

Nursing Implications

Dose adjustment in renal impairment. Can cause anaphylaxis, hemolytic anemia, and urticaria.

penicillin G (procaine preparations) (Wycillin, Crysticillin A.S.)

Indications

(antibiotic; penicillin, long-acting IM)
    Used to treat moderately severe infections and congenital syphilis.

Administration

Neonate:	50,000 units/kg/24 hr daily IM
Congenital syphilis:	50,000 units/kg/24 hr daily IM × 10 days
Infant or child:	25,000–50,000 units/kg/24 hr ÷ q12–24h IM (max. dose: 4.8 million units/24 hr)
Adult:	0.6–4.8 million units/24 hr ÷ q12–24h IM
Compatibility:	Sterile H_2O for injection

Nursing Implications

Do not give IV. May cause pain at IM injection site. If >1 day of treatment for congenital syphilis is missed, the whole course should be restarted. Side effects are similar to those in aqueous penicillin G, plus CNS stimulation and seizures.

penicillin V potassium (Pen•Vee K, V-Cillin K, and others)

Indications

(antibiotic; penicillin)

Used to treat mild to moderately severe bacterial infections of the upper respiratory tract, skin, and urinary tract; to treat group A streptococcal pharyngitis; and for prophylaxis of pneumococcal infections and rheumatic fever.

Administration

Child:	25–50 mg/kg/24 hr ÷ q6–8h PO (max. dose: 3 g/24 hr)
Adult:	250–500 mg/dose q6–8h PO
Acute group A streptococcal pharyngitis:	
Child:	250 mg b.i.d.–t.i.d. PO × 10 days
Adolescent or adult:	500 mg b.i.d.–t.i.d. PO × 10 days
Secondary rheumatic fever or pneumococcal prophylaxis:	
≤5 yr:	125 mg b.i.d. PO
>5 yr:	250 mg b.i.d. PO

Nursing Implications

Better GI absorption than penicillin G. Can cause rash, nausea, vomiting, diarrhea, and black hairy tongue. Best taken 1 hr before or 2 hr after meals, but can be taken with meals to decrease GI upset.

phenobarbital (Luminal, Solfoton, and others)

Indications

(barbiturate)

Used as anticonvulsant in grand mal, partial, and febrile seizures. Also used for sedation and for prevention and treatment of neonatal hyperbilirubinemia.

Administration

Sedation:	
Child:	6 mg/kg/24 hr ÷ t.i.d. PO
Adult:	30–120 mg/24 hr PO ÷ b.i.d.–t.i.d.

Preoperative sedation:
    Child: 1–3 mg/kg/dose IV/IM/PO 60–90 min before procedure

Status epilepticus:
    Loading dose IV:
        Neonate, infant, or child: 15–20 mg/kg in single or divided dose; may give additional 5-mg/kg doses q15–30min to max. dose of 30 mg/kg

    Maintenance dose PO/IV:
        Neonate: 3–5 mg/kg/24 hr ÷ daily–b.i.d.
        Infant: 5–6 mg/kg/24 hr ÷ daily–b.i.d.
        1–5 yr: 6–8 mg/kg/24 hr ÷ daily–b.i.d.
        6–12 yr: 4–6 mg/kg/24 hr ÷ daily–b.i.d.
        >12 yr: 1–3 mg/kg/24 hr ÷ daily–b.i.d.

Hyperbilirubinemia:
    <12 yr: 3–8 mg/kg/24 hr ÷ daily–b.i.d.

IV dilution:
    Direct IV: 1 mg/kg/min (max. dose: 30 mg/min for infant/child; 60 mg/min for adult >60 kg)
    Infusion: 2 mg/kg/min over 20–30 min

Compatibility: D_5W, NS, LR, $D_{10}W$

Nursing Implications

IV administration may cause respiratory arrest or hypotension. Side effects include drowsiness, cognitive impairment, ataxia, hypotension, hepatitis, rash, respiratory depression, and apnea. Can also cause hyperactivity, irritability, and insomnia as paradoxical reaction in children. Therapeutic levels: 15–40 mg/L.

phenytoin (Dilantin)
Indications

(anticonvulsant; class 1b antiarrhythmic)

Used in treatment and prevention of grand mal and complex partial seizures. Also used to treat ventricular arrhythmias associated with digitalis intoxication, prolonged Q-T interval, and surgical repair of congenital heart diseases.

Administration

Status epilepticus:
    Loading dose (all ages):   15–20 mg/kg/dose IV (max. dose: 1,500 mg/24 hr)

Maintenance for
   seizure disorders:
     Neonate: 5–8 mg/kg/24 hr ÷ q8–12h PO/IV
     Infant or child: Start 5 mg/kg/24 hr ÷ b.i.d.–t.i.d. PO/IV
       Usual ranges:
         6 mo–3 yr: 8–10 mg/kg/24 hr b.i.d.–t.i.d. PO/IV
         4–6 yr: 7.5–9 mg/kg/24 hr b.i.d.–t.i.d. PO/IV
         7–9 yr: 7–8 mg/kg/24 hr b.i.d.–t.i.d. PO/IV
         10–16 yr: 6–7 mg/kg/24 hr b.i.d.–t.i.d. PO/IV
     Adult: Start with 100 mg/dose q8h PO/IV
     Range: 300–600 mg/24 hr *or* 6–7 mg/kg/24 hr ÷
                     q8–24h PO/IV
Anti-arrhythmia:
   Loading dose (all ages): 1.25 mg/kg q5min IV up to total of 15 mg/kg
   Maintenance:
     Child: 5–10 mg/kg/24 hr ÷ q12h PO/IV
     Adult: 250 mg q.i.d. PO × 1 day, then 250 mg
                     q12h × 2 days, then 300–400 mg/24 hr ÷
                     q6–24h
IV dilution:
   Direct IV: Not to exceed 0.5 mg/kg/min in neonates,
                     1–3 mg/kg/min in others for max. rate of
                     50 mg/min. Flush with NS.
   Intermittent IV: Dilute with NS to <6 mg/mL
   Compatibility: NS only

Nursing Implications

Crystallizes with dextrose. Contraindicated in patients with heart block or sinus bradycardia. IM route not recommended. Assess for irritation and necrosis with IV use. Therapeutic levels for seizure disorders: 10–20 mg/L. Side effects include gingival hyperplasia, hirsutism, dermatitis, blood dyscrasias, ataxia, Stevens-Johnson syndrome, lymphadenopathy, liver damage, and nystagmus. Many drug interactions, so check insert or with pharmacist.

piperacillin (Pipracil)

Indications

(antibiotic; extended spectrum penicillin)

   Used in treatment of serious infections of skin, bone, joint, respiratory tract, and urinary tract. Often used for patients with CF. Also used to treat intraabdominal and gynecologic infections. Primary use is in treatment of serious carbenicillin- or ticarcillin-resistant *Pseudomonas aeruginosa* infections.

Administration

Neonate:

≤7 days, ≤36 wk gestation:	150 mg/kg/24 hr ÷ q12h IV
>36 wk gestation:	225 mg/kg/24 hr ÷ q8h IV
>7 days, ≤36 wk gestation:	225 mg/kg/24 hr ÷ q8h IV
>36 wk gestation:	300 mg/kg/24 hr ÷ q6h IV
Infant or child:	200–300 mg/kg/24 hr ÷ 4–6h IV/IM (max. dose: 24 g/24 hr)
CF:	300–600 mg/kg/24 hr ÷ q4–6h IV/IM (max. dose: 24 g/24 hr)
Adult:	2–4 g/dose q4–6h IV *or* 1–2 g/dose q6h IM (max. dose: 24 g/24 hr)

IV dilution:

Direct IV:	200 mg/mL over 3–5 min
Intermittent IV:	≤20 mg/mL over 30–60 min
Compatibility:	D$_5$W, NS, LR

Nursing Implications

May cause seizures, myoclonus, and fever. Assess IV site for irritation and phlebitis. Administer IM dose deep in a large muscle. If child is also receiving IV aminoglycosides, separate infusions by ≥2 hr.

potassium chloride (Many brands)

Indications

(KCl supplements)

Used to correct or prevent potassium deficiency.

Administration

Normal daily
requirements:

Neonate or infant:	2–6 mEq/kg/24 hr IV/PO
Child:	2–3 mEq/kg/24 hr IV/PO
Adult:	40–80 mEq/24 hr IV/PO

Hypokalemia:

Child:	1–4 mEq/kg/24 hr ÷ b.i.d.–q.i.d. PO 0.5–1 mEq/dose given as infusion of 0.5 mEq/kg/hr × 1–2 hr (max. IV infusion rate: 1 mEq/kg/hr in critical situations)
Adult:	40–100 mEq/24 hr ÷ b.i.d.–q.i.d. PO 10–20 mEq/dose to infuse over 2–3 hr (max. IV infusion rate: 40 mEq/hr)

IV dilution: Max. peripheral IV solution concentration: 40 mEq/L
                          Max. concentration for CVL: 150–200 mEq/L
                          Do not give IV push.

Compatibility: D₅W, NS, LR

Nursing Implications

Rapid IV infusion can cause arrhythmias. PO administration may cause GI disturbance and ulceration. Oral liquid should be diluted in water or juice. Monitor potassium levels.

prednisone (Deltasone and others)

Indications

(corticosteroid)

Used in management of adrenocortical insufficiency and for anti-inflammatory and immunosuppressant effects.

Administration

Anti-inflammatory or
   immunosuppressive: 0.5–2 mg/kg/24 hr ÷ daily–b.i.d. PO
Acute asthma: 2 mg/kg/24 hr daily–b.i.d. PO × 5 days (max.
                          dose: 80 mg/24 hr)

Nephrotic syndrome:
   Initial: 2 mg/kg/24 hr PO (max. dose: 80 mg/24 hr)

Nursing Implications

Doses must be tapered gradually to discontinue unless used ≤5 days. Further doses in nephrotic syndrome are individualized by nephrologist. Side effects include mood changes, seizures, hyperglycemia, diarrhea, nausea, and GI bleeding. Patients can have cushingoid effects and cataracts with prolonged use. Barbiturates, carbamazepine, phenytoin, rifampin, and INH may reduce effects of prednisone, whereas estrogens may enhance effects. Administer after meals or with food to decrease GI upset.

promethazine (Phenergan, Provigan, and others)

Indications

(antihistamine; antiemetic; phenothiazine derivative)

Used in symptomatic treatment of allergic conditions and motion sickness, as preoperative sedative, and for prevention and treatment of nausea and vomiting.

Administration

Antihistaminic:

Child:	0.1 mg/kg/dose q6h PO and 0.5 mg/kg/dose q.h.s. p.r.n. PO
Adult:	12.5 mg t.i.d. PO and 25 mg q.h.s. PO

Sedation:

Child:	0.5–1.1 mg/kg/dose q6h p.r.n. PO/PR/IV/IM
Adult:	25–50 mg/dose q4–6h p.r.n. PO/PR/IV/IM

Nausea and
  vomiting:

Child:	0.25–1 mg/kg/dose q4–6h p.r.n. PO/PR/IV/IM
Adult:	12.5–25 mg q4–6h p.r.n. PO/PR/IV/IM
Motion sickness:	First dose 0.5–1 hr before departure
Child:	0.5 mg/kg/dose q12h p.r.n. PO
Adult:	25 mg b.i.d. p.r.n. PO
IV dilution:	Undiluted 25 mg/mL no faster than 25 mg/min
Compatibility:	D_5W, NS, LR, $D_{10}W$

Nursing Implications

Observe for excessive sedation. Monitor BP, pulse, and respirations with IV use. IM administration preferred. Administer with food or milk to decrease GI distress. May cause profound sedation, blurred vision, and dystonic reactions.

ranitidine (Zantac)

Indications

(histamine-2 antagonist)

Used in prevention and treatment of duodenal ulcers and in management of GE reflux.

Administration

Neonate:	2–4 mg/kg/24 hr ÷ q8–12h PO
	2 mg/kg/24 hr ÷ q6–8h IV
Infant or child:	4–5 mg/kg/24 hr ÷ q8–12h PO (max. dose: 6 mg/ kg/24 hr)
	2–4 mg/kg/24 hr ÷ q6–8h IV/IM
Adult:	150 mg/dose b.i.d. *or* 300 mg/dose q.h.s. PO
	50 mg/dose q6–8h IV/IM (max. dose: 400 mg/ 24 hr)
Continuous infusion (all ages):	Administer daily IV dose over 24 hr

IV dilution:
    Direct IV: 2.5 mg/mL over 5 min
    Intermittent infusion
       (preferred):   0.5 mg/mL over 15–30 min
    Compatibility: D_5W, NS, LR, $D_{10}W$

Nursing Implications

Rapid infusion can cause bradycardia, tachycardia, or premature ventricular contractions. Can be added to total parenteral nutrition. Can cause headache, GI disturbances, malaise, insomnia, sedation, arthralgia, and hepatotoxicity. Antacids decrease absorption.

salmeterol (Serevent)

Indications

(bronchodilator)
    Used as maintenance of asthma and prevention of exercise-induced bronchospasm.

Administration

    Children > 12 yr: 2 inhalations b.i.d.
    Children 4–12 yr: 1 inhalation b.i.d.

Nursing Implications

If using to prevent exercise-induced bronchospasm, advise patient to use at least 30–60 minutes prior to exercise. Headache is a frequent side effect. Not for relief of acute episodes of bronchospasm.

spironolactone (Aldactone)

Indications

(diuretic, potassium sparing)
    Used in management of edema, hypertension, and primary hyperaldosteronism and in treatment of hirsutism.

Administration

Diuretic:
    Child: 1–3.3 mg/kg/24 hr ÷ b.i.d.–q.i.d. PO
    Adult: 25–200 mg/24 hr ÷ b.i.d.–q.i.d. PO (max. dose:
                    200 mg/24 hr)
Primary
    aldosteronism:
    Child: 125–325 mg/m^2/24 hr b.i.d.–q.i.d. PO

Adult: 400 mg daily PO × 4 days or 3–4 wk, then 100–400 mg
                     daily maintenance

Nursing Implications

Administer with food. Contraindicated in acute renal failure. May cause hyperkalemia, GI distress, rash, and gynecomastia. Potassium levels should be monitored.

sulfisoxazole (Gantrisin)

Indications

(antibiotic; sulfonamide derivative)

Used in treatment of UTIs, OM, and RF and for meningococcus prophylaxis.

Administration

Children ≥2 mo:
    Initial: 75 mg/kg/dose PO × 1
    Maintenance: 120–150 mg/kg/24 hr ÷ q4–6h PO (max. dose: 6 g/
                      24 hr)
Adult:
    Initial: 2–4 g × 1
    Maintenance: 4–8 g/24 hr ÷ q4–6h PO (max. dose: 8 g/24 hr)
OM prophylaxis: 50 mg/kg/dose q.h.s. PO
RF prophylaxis:
    <27 kg: 500 mg daily PO
    ≥27 kg: 100 mg daily PO
Meningococcus
  prophylaxis:
    <1 yr: 500 mg daily PO × 2 days
    1–12 yr: 500 mg b.i.d. PO × 2 days
    >12 yr: 1,000 mg b.i.d. PO × 2 days
Ophthalmic solution: 1–2 gtt. q1–4h

Nursing Implications

Give on empty stomach. Do not use in infants <2 mo of age. Contraindicated in urinary obstruction. Use with caution in renal or liver disease or G6PD deficiency. Maintain adequate fluid intake. Can cause HA, fever, rash, Stevens-Johnson syndrome, nausea, vomiting, and blood dyscrasias.

ticarcillin (Ticar)

Indications

(antibiotic; extended-spectrum penicillin)

Used in treatment of serious infections of skin, bone, joints, and urinary tract; acute and chronic respiratory tract infections; and septicemia. Often used to treat lung infections in children with CF.

Administration

Neonates:
≤7 days, <2 kg:	150 mg/kg/24 hr ÷ q12h IV/IM
≥2 kg:	225 mg/kg/24 hr ÷ q8h IV/IM
>7 days, <1.2 kg:	150 mg/kg/24 hr ÷ q12h IV/IM
1.2–2 kg:	225 mg/kg/24 hr ÷ q8h IV/IM
>2 kg:	300 mg/kg/24 hr ÷ q6–8h IV/IM

Infant or child:	200–300 mg/kg/24 hr ÷ q4–6h IV/IM (max. dose: 24 g/24 hr)
Adult:	1–4 g/dose q4–6h IV/IM
Uncomplicated UTIs:	
Child:	50–100 mg/kg/24 hr ÷ q6–8h IV/IM
Adult:	1 g/dose q6h IV/IM
CF:	300–600 mg/kg/24 hr ÷ q4–6h IV/IM (max. dose: 24 g/24 hr)
IV dilution:	100 mg/mL over 30–120 min; ≤50 mg/mL preferred
Compatibility:	D_5W, NS, LR

Nursing Implications

May cause decreased platelet aggregation, hypocalcemia, hypokalemia, hypernatremia, rash, hematuria, and increased aspartate aminotransferase. If child also receiving IV aminoglycosides, separate infusions by ≥2 hr.

ticarcillin/clavulanate (Timentin)

Indications

(antibiotic; extended-spectrum penicillin with β-lactamase inhibitor)

Same as ticarcillin except has β-lactamase inhibitor that broadens spectrum.

Administration

Doses based on ticarcillin; see ticarcillin (max. dose: 18–24 g/24 hr)

Nursing Implications

Same as ticarcillin.

tobramycin (Tobrex, Nebcin, TOBI, and others)

Indications

(antibiotic; aminoglycoside)

Used in treatment of serious gram-negative and staphylococcal infections when penicillin is contraindicated or gentamicin resistance has occurred. Also effective against *P. aeruginosa*. Used topically to treat ophthalmic infections and as inhalation therapy for management of CF patients with *P. aeruginosa*.

Administration

Neonate:	Dose depends on postconceptual and postnatal age and weight; consult pharmacology text
Child:	6–7.5 mg/kg/24 hr ÷ q8h IV/IM
CF:	7.5–10 mg/kg/24 hr ÷ q8h IV
Adult:	3–6 mg/kg/24 hr ÷ q8h IV/IM
Ophthalmic:	Apply thin ribbon of ointment to affected eye b.i.d.–t.i.d. *or* 1–2 gtt. of solution q4h
CF prophylaxis therapy (TOBI):	
≥6 yr–adult:	300 mg q12h in repeated cycles of 28 days on and 28 days off drug
IV dilution:	≤10 mg/mL over 30–60 min *or* direct injection over 15 min
Compatibility:	D_5W, NS

Nursing Implications

Therapeutic levels: peak: 6–10 mg/L (8–10 mg/L in pulmonary infections, neutropenia, and severe sepsis); trough: <2 mg/L. Can cause ototoxicity (effects synergistic with furosemide) and nephrotoxicity. Can also cause HA, rash, nausea, vomiting, weakness, and elevated liver enzymes.

When giving TOBI with other inhaled medicines, give it last. Separate IV administration from other antibiotics by ≥1 hr.

valproic acid/valproate sodium (Depakene, Depacon)

Indications

(anticonvulsant)

Used in management of simple and complex partial seizures, absence seizures, mixed seizure types, and myoclonic and grand mal seizures.

Administration

Initial:	10–15 mg/kg/24 hr ÷ daily–t.i.d. PO
Increment:	5–10 mg/kg/24 hr q wk (max. dose: 60 mg/kg/24 hr)
Maintenance:	30–60 mg/kg/24 hr ÷ b.i.d.–t.i.d. PO
IV:	Use same dose as PO ÷ q6h; convert back to PO as soon as possible
PR:	Use syrup diluted 1:1 with water; given PR as retention enema
Load:	20 mg/kg/dose
Maintenance:	10–15 mg/kg/dose q8h
IV dilution:	Dilute with ≥50 mL over 60 min (max. rate: 20 mg/min)
Compatibility:	D_5W, NS, LR

Nursing Implications

Contraindicated in hepatic disease. Can cause GI, blood, CNS, and liver toxicity; weight gain; transient alopecia; pancreatitis; nausea; vomiting; sedation; HA; and rash. Increases phenytoin, diazepam, and phenobarbital levels. Phenytoin, phenobarbital, and carbamazepine decrease valproic acid levels. Do not give syrup with carbonated beverages. Do not give tablet with milk. Therapeutic levels: 50–100 mg/L.

vancomycin (Vancocin and others)

Indications

(antibiotic)

Used in treatment of life-threatening infections such as endocarditis, meningitis, and osteomyelitis; in documented or suspected methicillin-resistant *Staphylococcus aureus*; and for infections associated with central lines, ventriculoperitoneal shunts, hemodialysis shunts, vascular grafts, and prosthetic heart valves. Used orally to treat staphylococcal enterocolitis or antibiotic-associated pseudomembranous colitis produced by *Clostridium difficile*.

Administration

Neonate:

<7 days, <1.2 kg:	10 mg/kg/dose q24h IV
1.2–2 kg:	10–15 mg/kg/dose q12–18h IV
>2 kg:	10–15 mg/kg/dose q8–12h IV
≥7 days, <1.2 kg:	15 mg/kg/dose q24h IV
1.2–2 kg:	10–15 mg/kg/dose q8–12h IV
>2 kg:	15–20 mg/kg/dose q8h IV

Infant or child:

CNS infection:	60 mg/kg/24 hr ÷ q6h IV

Other:	40 mg/kg/24 hr ÷ q6–8h IV (max. dose: 1 g/dose)
Adult:	2 g/24 hr ÷ q6–12h IV
C. difficile colitis:	
Child:	40–50 mg/kg/24 hr ÷ q6h PO × 7–10 days (max. dose: 500 mg/24 hr)
Adult:	125 mg/dose q6h PO × 7–10 days
IV dilution:	5 mg/mL over 60 min
Compatibility:	D_5W, NS, LR, $D_{10}W$

Nursing Implications

"Red man syndrome" (red flushing of neck and head with intense pruritus) with too rapid infusion. May need to increase infusion time to 120 min. Can also cause tachycardia, hypotension, chills, and nausea. Ototoxicity and nephrotoxicity may occur and may be exacerbated with concurrent aminoglycoside use. Therapeutic levels: peak: 25–40 mg/L; trough: <10 mg/L. Controversial whether levels need to be monitored.

DRUG ADMINISTRATION

IV Fluid Dilution and Rate Calculations

Determining Proper Dilution

Recommended dilution of a particular drug is 10 mg/mL.
Patient's dose is 500 mg IV q6h.

To determine the amount of fluid needed to dilute a particular drug, use the following equation:

$$\frac{10 \text{ mg}}{1 \text{ mL}} = \frac{500 \text{ mg}}{x \text{ mL}} \text{ (Cross multiply)}$$

$$10x = 500$$

$$x = 50 \text{ mL}$$

So you will dilute 500 mg in 50 mL to get the proper concentration of 10 mg/mL.

Determining Proper Rate

Many IV pumps can be set for volume and time, so this step may not be necessary.

$$\frac{\text{volume to be infused} \times \text{drip factor}}{\text{time (min)}} = \text{drops (gtt.)/min}$$

Example: We want to dilute the aforementioned drug in 50 mL and give over 30 min. Drip factor in pediatric clients is usually 60 because of use of microdrips.

$$\frac{50 \text{ mL} \times 60}{30 \text{ min}} = \frac{3,000}{30}$$

= 100 gtt./min or with drip factor of 60 drops/mL, is also 30 min. 100 mL/hr

Syringe pumps can be set for amount to be infused and for time.

Safe Drug Calculations

Determine child's weight in kilograms.
    Example: Child weighs 22 pounds.

$$22 \text{ pounds} \div 2.2 \text{ pounds/kg} = 10 \text{ kg}$$

Recommended safe dose is 200–400 mg/kg/24 hr q6h.
    Calculate 200 mg $\times$ 10 kg and 400 mg $\times$ 10 kg to get safe range for 24 hr. Safe range 2,000–4,000 mg/24 hr. Divide by 4 to get safe range for each dose given q6h. Safe dose range is 500–1,000 mg/dose.
    The aforementioned drug comes in a solution of 1,000 mg/mL. We want to give a dose of 500 mg. To calculate the amount to draw up, use the following equation:

$$\frac{1,000 \text{ mg}}{1 \text{ mL}} = \frac{500 \text{ mg}}{x \text{ mL}} \text{ (Cross multiply)}$$

$$1,000x = 500$$

$$x = 0.5 \text{ mL}$$

Preparation for Drug Administration

General Guidelines

- Start with clean area.
- Verify MD/APRN medication order.
- Obtain proper drug and proper strength.
- Assemble needed equipment.
- Draw up medication or check unit dose.
- Make sure you have the necessary supplies (e.g., alcohol swab, bandages, proper needle for IV system, label, nipple, syringe, cup, drink) before entering client's room.
- Take med sheet or card to compare with client's identification band.
- Know how client has taken and tolerated medications previously (e.g., Can client swallow pills? Can client tolerate volume?)
- Do not give medications in playroom. It is a safe area. Take child out of playroom to administer any medication.

- Be truthful; let child know what to expect. Explain child and caregiver roles. Try not to let caregiver threaten child. Encourage caregivers to comfort only.

Infants	Need TLC before and after.
Toddlers	Need immediate preparation. Do not offer unreal choices. Allow caregiver to help with oral medications.
Preschool children	Need to know what they are expected to do. Let them handle equipment. A bandage is very important for body integrity.
School-age children	Need explanation of their role and choices when possible. Longer preparation time needed for invasive procedures.
Adolescents	Generally want more information. Privacy is important. Preserve "tough" image. Recognize need for independence. Allow client choices (e.g., site), if appropriate.

Administration

Seven Rights
Right drug
Right dose
Right time
Right route
Right client
Right reason
Right documentation

Oral Medications
Crush tablets and mix with small amount of hot water and then syrup. Do not mix in large volumes or add to infant's bottle. Be aware of taste. Syrups are sweet, elixirs are bitter. Use cup, spoon, syringe, nipple (with syrups only) as appropriate for client. Give slowly. If using syringe, place it halfway back at side of tongue. Remember normal tongue thrust is present until 4–5 mo.

Intramuscular (IM)

Site	Comment
Vastus lateralis	Most medications
Ventro gluteal	Not until 3 yr; check hospital policy
Deltoid	Less invasive; usually not used until 3 yr; use with nonirritating medications

Age	Amount
Birth–3 yr	1 mL
3–6 yr	1.5 mL
6–15 yr	1.5–2 mL
Adult	2–3 mL

Age	Needle size
Birth–4 mo	5/8 inch
4 mo–10 yr	1 inch
10 yr–adult	$1^1/_2$ inch

Use smallest gauge needle possible; larger gauges may be needed for viscous medications and to prevent bending.

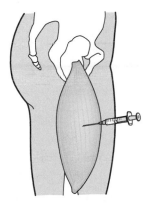

Vastus lateralis

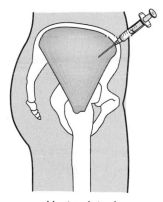

Ventrogluteal

Preferred Intramuscular Injection Sites in Children

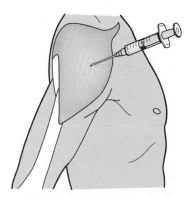

Deltoid

Preferred Intramuscular Injection Sites in Children

Subcutaneous (SC)

Sites   Same as IM
Amount   0.5 mL
Needle size 5/8–1 inch

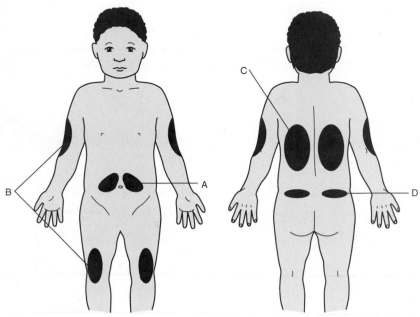

Subcutaneous Injection Sites: A. Abdomen; B. Lateral and Anterior Aspects of Upper Arm and Thigh; C. Scapular Area of Back; D. Upper Ventrodorsal Gluteal Area

Intravenous (IV)

Follow guidelines for proper dilution and time.

Check IV site for patency before and during infusion.

Check to be sure site and needle size are adequate for volume to be administered.

Flush IV tubing at same rate as medication administration to make sure all medication has been administered.

Rectal

Is invasive to most ages. Have preschoolers "pant like a puppy dog" to relax sphincter. May need to hold buttock cheeks together to prevent expelling. If you need to divide suppository to get correct dose, do so lengthwise to allow for easier insertion and to get better distribution of medication.

Nasogastric (NG) or Gastrostomy Tube (GT)

Check for placement before administering medications. Research has demonstrated that this is most accurately assessed by testing the pH of the gastric aspirate; an acidic reading should be determined. If aspirate pH >5, a chest X ray should be performed to confirm placement. Be sure to crush pills well and flush with water to prevent clogging tube.

Topical

Apply thin layer because of increased skin permeability.

Diaper can act as occlusive dressing and cause increased absorption of medication.

Eye

Put drops in the inner canthus. Put ointment in the lower lid. Tell the child that the ointment will blur vision. If the child will not cooperate, place the drops in the inner canthus and hold the head still so he or she cannot turn to the side. When the child opens his or her eyes to see why you have not gone away, the medication will go into the eyes. Apply pressure to the puncta at the inner aspect of the lower lid for 1 min to help prevent medication from going into nasopharynx.

Ear

In children <3 yr, pull the pinnae down and back to straighten the ear canal. If >3 yr, pull the pinnae up and back. Try to keep the child on his or her side for 1 min after administration if possible. Make sure medication is warmed to at least room temperature.

Nasal

Tip the head back and keep back for 1 min after administration of drops if possible to prevent strangling sensation of medication running into the posterior pharynx. Remember to sit the child up for administration of nasal sprays so they will properly aerosolize.

Immunization Schedule

Recommended childhood and adolescent immunization schedule,[1] by vaccine and age–United States, 2005

Vaccine	Birth	1 mo	2 mos	4 mos	6 mos	12 mos	15 mos	18 mos	24 mos	4–6 yrs	11–12 yrs	13–18 yrs
Hepatitis B[2]	HepB#1 only if mother HBsAg (–)	HepB #2			HepB #3						HepB series	
Diphtheria, tetanus, pertussis[3]			DTaP	DTaP	DTaP			DTaP		DTaP	Td	Td
Haemophilus influenzae type b[4]			Hib	Hib	Hib[4]	Hib						
Inactivated poliovirus			IPV	IPV	IPV		IPV			IPV		
Measles, mumps, rubella[5]						MMR #1				MMR #2	MMR #2	
Varicella[6]						Varicella				Varicella		
Pneumococcal[7]			PCV	PCV	PCV	PCV	PCV		PCV	PPV		
Influenza[8]					Influenza (yearly)					Influenza (yearly)		
Hepatitis A[9]										Hepatitis A series		

Vaccines below red line are for selected populations

☐ Range of recommended ages ☐ Catch-up immunization ☐ Preadolescent assessment

1. This schedule indicates the recommended ages for routine administration of currently licensed childhood vaccines, as of December 1, 2004, for children aged ≤18 years. Any dose not administered at the recommended age should be administered at any subsequent visit when indicated and feasible. ▮ Indicates age groups that warrant special effort to administer those vaccines not previously administered. Additional vaccines might be licensed and recommended during the year. Licensed combination vaccines may be used whenever any components of the combination are indicated and other components of the vaccine are not contra indicated. Providers should consult package inserts for detailed recommendations. Clinically significant adverse events that follow immunization should be reported to the Vaccine Adverse Event Reporting System; guidance is available at http://www.vaers.org or by telephone, 800-822-7967.

2. Hepatitis B (HepB) vaccine. All infants should receive the first dose of HepB vaccine soon after birth and before hospital discharge; the first dose may also be administered by age 2 months if the mother is hepatitis B surface antigen (HBsAg) negative. Only monovalent HepB may be used for the birth dose. Monovalent or combination vaccine containing HepB may be used to complete the series. Four doses of vaccine may be administered when a birth dose is administered. The second dose should be administered at least 4 weeks after the first dose, except for combination vaccines, which cannot be administered before age 6 weeks. The third dose should be administered at least 16 weeks after the first dose and at least 8 weeks after the second dose. The final dose in the vaccination series (third or fourth dose) should not be administered before age 24 weeks. *Infants born to HBsAg-positive mothers* should receive HepB and 0.5 mL of hepatitis B immune globulin (HBIG) at separate sites within 12 hours of birth. The second dose is recommended at age 1–2 months. The final dose in the immunization series should not be administered before age 24 weeks. These infants should be tested for HBsAg and antibody to HBsAg at age 9–15 months. *Infants born to mothers whose HBsAg status is unknown* should receive the first dose of the HepB series within 12 hours of birth. Maternal blood should be drawn as soon as possible to determine the mother's HBsAg status; if the HBsAg test is positive, the infant should receive HBIG as soon as possible (no later than age 1 week). The second dose is recommended at age 1–2 months. The last dose in the immunization series should not be administered before age 24 weeks.

3. Diphtheria and tetanus toxoids and acellular pertussis (DTaP) vaccine. The fourth dose of DTaP may be administered as early as age 12 months, provided 6 months have elapsed since the third dose and the child is unlikely to return at age 15–18 months. The final dose in the series should be administered at age ≥4 years. Tetanus and diphtheria toxoids (Td) is recommended at age 11–12 years if at least 5 years have elapsed since the last dose of tetanus and diphtheria toxoid-containing vaccine. Subsequent routine Td boosters are recommended every 10 years.

4. Haemophilus influenzae type b (Hib) conjugate vaccine. Three Hib conjugate vaccines are licensed for infant use. If PRP-OMP (PedvaxHIB® or ComVax® [Merck]) is administered at ages 2 and 4 months, a dose at age 6 months is not required. DTaP/Hib combination products should not be used for primary immunization in infants at ages 2, 4, or 6 months but can be used as boosters after any Hib vaccine. The final dose in the series should be administered at age ≥12 months.

(Continued)

Recommended childhood and adolescent immunization schedule,[1] by vaccine and age—United States, 2005 (*Continued*)

5. Measles, mumps, and rubella (MMR) vaccine. The second dose of MMR is recommended routinely at age 4–6 years but may be administered during any visit provided at least 4 weeks have elapsed since the first dose and both doses are administered beginning at or after age 12 months. Those who have not previously received the second dose should complete the schedule by age 11–12 years.

6. Varicella vaccine. Varicella vaccine is recommended at any visit at or after age 12 months for susceptible children (i.e., those who lack a reliable history of chickenpox). Susceptible persons aged ≥13 years should receive 2 doses administered at least 4 weeks apart.

7. Pneumococcal vaccine. The heptavalent pneumococcal conjugate vaccine (PCV) is recommended for all children aged 2–23 months and for certain children aged 24–59 months. The final dose in the series should be administered at age ≥12 months. Pneumococcal polysaccharide vaccine (PPV) is recommended in addition to PCV for certain groups at high risk. See *MMWR* 2000; 49(No. RR-9).

8. Influenza vaccine. Influenza vaccine is recommended annually for children aged ≥6 months with certain risk factors (including, but not limited to, asthma, cardiac disease, sickle cell disease, human immunodeficiency virus [HIV], and diabetes); health-care workers, and other persons (including household members) in close contact with persons in groups at high risk (see *MMWR* 2004;53[No. RR-6]). In addition, healthy children aged 6–23 months and close contacts of healthy children aged 0–23 months are recommended to receive influenza vaccine because children in this age group are at substantially increased risk for influenza-related hospitalizations. For healthy persons aged 5–49 years, the intranasally administered, live, attenuated influenza vaccine (LAIV) is an acceptable alternative to the intramuscular trivalent inactivated influenza vaccine (TIV). See *MMWR* 2004;53(No. RR-6). Children receiving TIV should be administered a dosage appropriate for their age (0.25 mL if aged 6–35 months or 0.5 mL if aged ≥3 years). Children aged ≤8 years who are receiving influenza vaccine for the first time should receive 2 doses (separated by at least 4 weeks for TIV and at least 6 weeks for LAIV).

9. Hepatitis A vaccine. Hepatitis A vaccine is recommended for children and adolescents in selected states and regions and for certain groups at high risk; consult your local public health authority. Children and adolescents in these states, regions, and groups who have not been immunized against hepatitis A can begin the hepatitis A immunization series during any visit. The 2 doses in the series should be administered at least 6 months apart. See *MMWR* 1999;48(No. RR-12).

CHAPTER 5

ESSENTIAL CLINICAL SKILLS

PERFORMING CARDIOPULMONARY RESUSCITATION (CPR)

I. Airway (most pediatric arrests are respiratory events)
   A. Determine unresponsiveness
   B. Activate emergency medical service
   C. Observe for obstruction, which is the most common precipitating event in arrest
   D. Clear oropharynx of secretions or vomitus
   E. Open airway
      1. Tilt head and lift chin
      2. Thrust jaw
      3. Maintain cervical spine alignment: do not hyperextend neck
      4. Insert oral or nasal airway to prevent airway obstruction

II. Breathing
   A. Determine breathlessness (look, listen, feel for breathing for 3–5 sec)
   B. Ventilate using bag-valve mask until placement of ETT or mouth-to-mouth is used in the field
   C. Give 2 slow rescue breaths with force sufficient to raise chest
   D. If airway obstructed, reposition and reattempt rescue breaths
      1. 5 abdominal thrusts (children >1 yr old)
      2. 5 back blows (children <1 yr old)
      3. 5 chest thrusts (children <1 yr old)
      4. Tongue-jaw lift and finger sweep in children >8 yr (in children <8 yr, finger sweep only if foreign object is visible)
   E. Rescue breathing only (pulse present)
      1. Children <8 yr old: 1 breath q 3 sec (approximately 20 per min)
      2. Children >8 yr old: 1 breath q 4 sec (approximately 15 per min)

III. Circulation
  A. Palpate pulse after rescue breaths for 5–10 seconds
    1. Carotid in children >1 yr old
    2. Brachial in children <1 yr old
  B. If pulse is absent, begin chest compressions (need firm surface)
    1. Find chest landmarks
      a. Child >1 yr old: lower sternum, 2 fingerbreaths above sternal notch
      b. Child <1 yr old: 1 fingerbreath below intersection of sternum and imaginary line between nipples (be sure fingers are not over xiphoid process)
    2. Compression rate
      a. Children <1 yr old: 100 per min
      b. Children 1–8 yr old: 100 per min
      c. Children >8 yr old: 80–100 per min
    3. Compression-breath ratio
      a. Children <1 yr old: 1 breath; 5 compressions
      b. Children 1–8 yr old: 1 breath; 5 compressions
      c. Children >8 yr old: 2 breaths; 15 compressions
    4. Compression depth
      a. Children <1 yr old: 1/2–1 inch
      b. Children 1–8 yr old: 1–1½ inches
      c. Children >8 yr old: 1½–2 inches

Recent studies have documented the benefits of caregiver presence during CPR. The Emergency Nurses Association supports the option of family presence during resuscitation efforts. Be familiar with your institution's policies and procedures on caregiver presence during resuscitation.

INFECTION CONTROL

Standard precautions for infection control are designed to reduce the risk of transmission of bloodborne and other pathogens. There are five main routes of transmission: contact, droplet, airborne, common vehicle, and vectorborne. Standard precaution guidelines are designed to interrupt the mode of transmission. Standard precautions involve the use of barrier protection, such as gloves, goggles, gown, and masks, to prevent contamination from blood, all body fluids, secretions and excretions (except sweat), nonintact skin, and mucous membranes. Standard precautions are designed for *all* clients to reduce the risk of transmission for both recognized and unrecognized infection sources.

The following basic principles should be observed:

- Wash hands between clients and after contact with blood, body fluids, secretions, and excretions and after contact with articles or equipment contaminated by them.

- Wash hands immediately after removal of gloves.
- Wear gloves when touching blood, body fluids, secretions, excretions, nonintact skin, mucous membranes, or contaminated articles.
- Remove gloves and wash hands between client care.
- If client-care activities can generate splashes or sprays of blood or body fluids, wear masks, eye protection, or face shields.
- Wear a gown if soiling of clothes from blood or body fluids is likely.
- Wash hands after removal of gown.
- Clean equipment between client use and discard single-use items.
- Keep contaminated linens in leak-proof bags and handle in a manner to prevent skin and mucous-membrane exposure.
- Discard sharp instruments and needles in a puncture-resistant container. The Centers for Disease Control and Prevention (CDC) recommends that needles be uncapped for disposal or capped by use of a mechanical device.
- Determine reason for isolation and mode of transmission.

Isolation Category

- *Airborne precautions* apply to clients with known or suspected infections transmittable by the airborne route (e.g., measles, varicella, tuberculosis [TB]); special air handling and ventilation required; client must be in private room; mask or respiratory protection device is necessary
- *Droplet precautions* apply to clients with known or suspected infections transmittable by the droplet route (e.g., *H. influenzae* infections [meningitis, pneumonia, epiglottitis, sepsis, diphtheria, mycoplasm pneumonia, pertussis, scarlet fever, rubella]); droplets are generated during sneezing, coughing, and talking; special air handling and ventilation are not required; place in private room or with cohort clients; masks are necessary
- *Contact precautions* are used to reduce the risk of transmission by direct or indirect contact; apply to clients with GI, respiratory, skin, or wound infections, RSV; place in private room or with cohort clients; gloves, gowns, and masks (if spraying possible) are necessary

Isolation for TB

- TB isolation practices should be used in all clients with known or suspected TB.
- Client should be placed in a negative airflow private room with door closed.
- Health care workers must use a high-efficiency particulate air (HEPA) respirator or an N95 particulate respirator mask when entering the room. Check institution policies for type of mask available, reusability, storage, and proper fitting requirements.

CLINICAL SKILLS AND TIPS

To Encourage Fluid Intake

Melt Popsicle in microwave until slushy. Child can then eat it with a spoon or straw. Provides relief for sore throats. Offer a 5- to 10-cc syringe. Show child how to draw up liquid and squirt it in his or her mouth. Works best with 3–10 yr olds. Improves intake because it is fun. Can also give child a small medicine cup to drink from. Involve parents to encourage child's cooperation.

To Encourage Deep Breathing

Have child blow bubbles or a pinwheel. Can have child "blow out the light" with a pen light. Have child blow a cotton ball across the bedside table into a paper cup and pretend it is a soccer or hockey goal. Pretend that child is blowing out candles on a cake.

To Decrease Gagging

Gently press back on the chin to help stop gag reflex. Works best in young infants.

To Calm Fussy Babies

If you have ensured baby is not hungry nor needs changing, check to be sure IV has not infiltrated. This is the most common cause of inconsolable fussy babies. Expose IV as much as necessary to ensure patency. Compare extremities for size and shape to determine swelling. If IV is patent, try rocking motions, soothing voice, singing, or playing music to calm baby.

To Start IV in Infants

Best site for young infants is the head. It causes less restriction in movement and the least amount of disturbance in achievement of developmental tasks. Infants forget it is there and leave it alone. If it infiltrates, there is little tissue damage because circulation to area is less impaired than in the extremities. When the scalp is used, save a lock of the infant's hair that is shaved for the caregiver to put in the baby book to remember first "hair cut." This helps ease caregiver's chagrin over infant having his or her head shaved.

Warm Soaks

Warm soaks to extremities stay warm longer if extremity is wrapped in a warm wash cloth and then "diapered" with a disposable diaper. The plastic helps keep warmth in longer and keeps bed from getting wet.

SPECIMEN COLLECTION TIPS
Urine Collection
Infants

Clean area and allow to dry. Prepare area with Benzoin if skin is intact, let dry until sticky, and attach pediatric urine bag. Can extract urine from bag with small-gauge needle and leave bag attached if more urine is needed. Young infants have a reflex that, if they are suspended supine on the nurse's hand, he or she can press at base of spine and gently stroke upward with two fingers. This causes infant to arch back, raise buttocks in the air, cry, and void if bladder is full. Allows for quick collection of specimen in bag or cup held under infant.

Toddlers or Preschoolers

Place hat-type specimen collection container in the hole in child's potty chair. Then child can void normally and not have to "perform" by voiding in a cup.

School-Age Children or Adolescents

Easier to collect clean-catch specimen if he or she sits backward on toilet. This makes child spread his or her legs for cleaning and to hold the cup.

Stool Collection

If you need to collect loose stool in infants to send for electrolytes, you can bag the anus using a pediatric urine bag. You may want to put plastic wrap in the diaper to use to scrape stool for collection.

Blood Collection

Warm extremity before capillary draws. Wipe area with alcohol again after the stick to increase blood flow. Squeezing extremity or digit can increase hemolysis and artificially elevate potassium results. Capillary hematocrit (Hct) can be 5%–10% higher than venous Hct. For venous collections, antecubital vein is best for all age groups and hurts less than using veins on hand or foot.

ADMINISTRATION OF OXYGEN
NIC Intervention Label and Definition (3320): Oxygen Therapy—Administration of Oxygen and Monitoring of Its Effectiveness

Because oxygen is considered a medication, a physician order containing the concentration, flow rate, and delivery device is necessary. Method of delivery selected is based on the required oxygen concentration and child's ability to cooperate.

Types of oxygen delivery devices include:

- Plastic hood
  - Used to deliver high concentration of oxygen (100%)
  - Safety considerations include preventing the hood from rubbing against skin on infant's face and shoulder

- Nasal cannula or nasal prongs
  - Used to deliver lower concentration of oxygen (50%)
  - Should not be used if greater than 4 lpm is required
  - Safety considerations include inspecting the nares for any irritation
  - Assess potential pressure sites at least q2hr
  - Best used with cooperative children

- Mask
  - Delivers 35%–60% oxygen at 6–10 lpm flow rates
  - Not well-tolerated by toddlers and young school-age children
  - Snugly fit child
  - Assess potential pressure sites at least q2hr

- Tent
  - Used with young children to provide concentration of oxygen between 30%–50%
  - Tent should be closed by keeping lower edges tucked underneath the crib or bed mattress
  - Avoid metal, battery-operated, or electrical toys
  - Child may require frequent changing of clothing and linen in order to keep child warm and dry while in oxygen tent
  - Use oxygen analyzer to determine oxygen concentration in tent

Procedure:

1. Verify orders for oxygen including flow rate, concentration, and delivery device.
2. SAFETY: Keep flammable or volatile solutions outside of room.
3. Attach flow meter to oxygen outlet and then secure delivery device to flow meter.
4. Attach humidification container (sterile water).
5. Involve parent(s) or other caregivers in preparing the child in order to enhance child's cooperation and reduce anxiety or fear.
6. Adjust flow meter appropriately in compliance with physician's order.
7. Assess child's response: respiratory rate, respiratory effort, breath sounds, pulse oximetry, skin color, HR, mental status.

USE OF RESTRAINTS
NIC Intervention Label and Definition (6580): Physical Restraint—Application, Monitoring, and Removal or Mechanical Restraining Devices or Manual Restraints, Which Are Used to Limit Physical Mobility of a Patient

Various restraints may be used to ensure child safety and facilitate the performance of procedures while promoting comfort. These include: therapeutic hugging (human restraint), mummy restraint, jacket restraint, elbow restraint, and arm or leg restraints. The Joint Commission on Accreditation of Healthcare Organizations (JCAHO) has established standards of care related to using restraints with children. A physician's order including type of restraint is necessary. Restraints are to be discontinued as soon as they are no longer needed.

Types of restraints include:

- Therapeutic hugging (human restraint)
  - Temporary holding position providing close physical contact
  - May be performed in sitting or supine position
  - Used to prevent child from moving during procedures

- Mummy restraint
  - Used as short-term restraint to prevent child from moving during procedures such as venipuncture
  - Blanket or sheet is used
  - Fold corner of blanket, placing child with folded edge at shoulders; fold blanket over arm, across abdomen, tucking edge behind back; repeat for left arm

- Jacket restraint
  - Used to prevent child from climbing out of crib or bed
  - Jacket is placed over child's clothing with ties in back
  - Secure ties to bed frame using half-bow knots

- Elbow restraint
  - Used to prevent child from bending elbow or reaching the head or face
  - Place restraint over child's clothing
  - Place restraint over each elbow and wrap snugly (but not too tight) being sure restraint does not rub wrist or axilla
  - Secure restraint using ties, Velcro, or tape (this will depend upon type used)

- Arm or leg restraint
  - o Used to immobilize extremity for procedures or treatment
  - o Cloth, clove-hitch, and gauze type restraints are available
  - o Place padding around wrist or ankle to prevent skin chafing
  - o Secure restraint to bed frame

Procedure:

1. Explain to the child and family why the restraint is necessary. Reassure child that restraint is not a punishment.
2. Restraining device should be removed and reapplied q1–2 hr.
3. Patient assessment should include skin beneath restraint, circulation, and sensation.
4. Restraints should *never* be tied to side rails.
5. Document use of restraints and patient assessment.

NASOTRACHEAL SUCTIONING

NIC Intervention Label and Definition (3160): Airway Suctioning—Removal of Airway Secretion by Inserting a Suction Catheter into the Patient's Oral Airway or Trachea

Nasotracheal suctioning during hospitalization is a sterile procedure performed to remove secretions from the child's airway. This procedure requires a physician's order.

DETERMINING ENDOTRACHEAL TUBE (ETT), SUCTION CATHETER, AND LARYNGOSCOPE BLADE SIZES

Age	Weight (in kg)	ETT Size	Suction Catheter	Laryngoscope Blade
Newborn	3	3.0–3.5	6 French	1
Infant	5	3.5–4.0	8 French	1
1 yr	10	4.0–4.5	8 French	1½
3 yr	15	4.5–5.0	8 French	2
6 yr	20	5.0–5.5	10 French	2
10 yr	30	6.0–6.5 cuffed	10 French	2
Adolescent	50	7.0–7.5 cuffed	10 French	3
Adult	70	7.5–8.0 cuffed	12–14 French	3

$$\text{Endotracheal tube diameter (mm)} = \frac{\text{age (years)} + 16}{4}$$

Procedure:

1. Wash hands.
2. Prepare child and family for procedure in order to enhance cooperation and reduce anxiety or fear.
3. Perform baseline assessment of respiratory status (i.e., RR, skin color, respiratory effort, breath sounds, oxygen saturation).
4. Open and prepare suction kit and normal saline.
5. Oxygenate child above baseline saturation as suctioning may cause hypoxia.
6. Wear mask, gloves, goggles, and gown in accordance with standard and droplet precautions (see agency policy).
7. Holding suction catheter with your dominant hand, connect it to the suction tubing with your nondominant hand. Check suction pressure once suction catheter is connected.
    a. Suction levels should be set as follows: 80–100 mm Hg for infants and children under 10 and 100 120 mm Hg for children 10 and over.
8. Determine correct distance to advance suction catheter by measuring from tip of child's nose to ear, noting position on the catheter.
9. Moisten catheter with sterile saline.
10. Using downward motion, advance catheter into the nare no farther than the premeasured distance.
11. Apply intermittent suctioning by covering the suction control hole with thumb. Rotate catheter while withdrawing.
12. Note color, amount, and consistency of secretions.
13. Suction time should be limited to no more than 5 seconds for infants and 15 seconds for children.
14. Reoxygenate the child to baseline saturation as suctioning may cause hypoxia.
15. Clear the catheter by flushing with normal saline.
16. Repeat steps 10–11 as needed to clear nasopharynx of secretions, allowing 30-second intervals between each episode of suctioning. Total suctioning time should be limited to no more than 5 minutes.
17. Reassess respiratory status to determine the effectiveness of the procedure (i.e., RR, skin color, respiratory effort, breath sounds, oxygen saturation).

TRACHEOSTOMY CARE

NIC Intervention Label and Definition (3180): Artificial Airway Management— Maintenance of Endotracheal and Tracheostomy Tubes and Preventing Complications Associated with Their Use

Tracheostomy care and dressing change should be done at least once per shift. It may be required more often if the site or dressing becomes soiled or wet. Spare tracheostomy tubes should be available directly at the bedside. For a new tracheostomy, spare tracheostomy tubes should be of the same size and half size smaller. For established tracheostomies, spare tracheostomy tubes should be the same size.

Procedure:

1. Wash hands.
2. Prepare the child and family for the procedure in order to enhance cooperation and reduce anxiety or fear.
3. Determine baseline respiratory assessment (i.e., RR, skin color, respiratory effort, breath sounds, oxygen saturation).
4. Wear mask, gloves, goggles, and gown in accordance with standard and droplet precautions (see agency policy).
5. Assemble supplies and equipment including preslit Sof-Wick dressing, cotton-tipped applicators, pipe cleaners, small hemostat, precut twill tape, sterile container, normal saline or sterile water, and ½-strength hydrogen peroxide.
6. Position child without hyperextending neck.
7. Preoxygenate child as needed in order to reduce chance of hypoxia during procedure.
8. Unlock inner cannula and inspect the integrity of the tracheostomy tube. Clean the trachestomy tube and cannula with soft-tipped applicators or pipe cleaners and rinse with sterile water.
9. Place cannula into container with hydrogen peroxide. Agitate for a couple of minutes. Allow cannula to air dry. Replace inner cannula and lock into place.
10. Remove the old dressing by gently lifting the tracheostomy tube flange.
11. Use cotton-tipped applicators moistened with ½-strength peroxide to clean around stoma site, moving outward from the stoma (avoid cleaning toward stoma). Use multiple applicators as needed to remove secretions.
12. Rinse area using cotton-tipped applicators soaked with normal saline or sterile water, again moving outward from the stoma.
13. Cleanse the area behind the flanges of the tracheostomy and around the neck with damp gauze.
14. Dry skin thoroughly using clean, dry applicators and gauze.
15. Place new Sof-Wick dressing under the tracheostomy tube flanges using hemostat and fingers.
16. Remove old trach ties from flange. Attach twill tape to flange and tie securely. Ties should be tight enough to prevent dislodgement but loose enough to fit one finger between tie and child's neck.
17. Reassess respiratory status and client response to procedure (i.e., RR, skin color, respiratory effort, breath sounds, oxygen saturation).

MEASURING PEAK EXPIRATORY FLOW RATE (PEFR)

NIC Intervention Label and Definition (3210): Asthma Management—Identification, Treatment, and Prevention of Reactions to Inflammation or Constriction in the Airway Passages

The measurement of PEFR has become a standard of care for children with asthma. PEFR represents how well air moves out of the child's lungs. Lower PEFRs are seen during acute exacerbations of asthma as a result of impaired expiration and air trapping during airway obstruction.

Procedure:

1. Wash hands.
2. Prepare the child and family for the procedure in order to enhance cooperation and reduce anxiety or fear.
3. Child should be sitting or standing to maximize lung expansion.
4. Child should place mouthpiece of meter in mouth, take deep breath, close lips around mouthpiece, and blow as fast and as hard as possible into mouthpiece.
5. Read number on meter.
6. After child rests 20–30 seconds between readings, have him or her repeat the process two or three more times.
7. Record highest (not average) reading.

CARE OF CENTRAL OR PERIPHERALLY INSERTED CENTRAL CATHETERS

NIC Intervention Label and Definition (4220): Peripherally Inserted Central (PIC) Catheter Care—Insertion and Maintenance of a Peripherally Inserted Central Catheter

A central venous catheter is an IV catheter that has been inserted into a large central vein, with the catheter tip in or near the right atrium. This type of IV access is often used with children needing long-term IV therapy, total parenteral nutrition, or chemotherapy. A variety of central line catheters are used in the clinical area (Broviac, Hickman, PICC). Central venous catheters require flushing, usually with heparinized saline. The catheter site is usually covered with transparent occlusive dressings that are changed under sterile procedure every 2–3 days depending upon agency policy.

Procedure:

1. Gather necessary equipment: mask, nonsterile gloves, sterile gloves, cleansing solution for site, dressing materials (prepackaged central venous line dressing kits are available).
2. Prepare the child and family for the procedure in order to enhance cooperation and reduce anxiety or fear.
3. Wash hands.
4. Put on mask and don nonsterile gloves. Remove old dressing.
5. Assess IV site for redness, swelling, and drainage.
6. Remove and discard nonsterile gloves. Wash hands.
7. Open supplies and set up sterile field.
8. Don sterile gloves.
9. Cleanse insertion site and surrounding area with solution (i.e., povidone-iodine, 70% alcohol, alcohol-acetone depending upon agency policy). Swab area beginning at catheter site and cleansing outward in circular pattern (without returning swab to center). This maintains asepsis by cleaning from least contaminated to most contaminated area.
10. Clean catheter last, moving from insertion site along catheter.
11. Apply skin prep to area avoiding ½-inch area directly around catheter exit site.
12. Apply ointment per agency policy.
13. Apply new sterile dressing (clear occlusive dressing).

ADMINISTERING NEBULIZED MEDICATIONS

NIC Intervention Label and Definition (2311): Medication Administration Inhalation–Preparing and Administering Inhaled Medications

Some medications are aerosolized by a nebulizer into a fine mist and directly delivered into the lungs. Absorption from this route is fast and noninvasive. Nebulized medications are often used to treat children with respiratory distress.

Procedure:

1. Verify physician order for nebulized medication.
2. Prepare the child and family for the procedure in order to enhance cooperation and reduce anxiety or fear.

3. Wash hands and prepare medication.
4. Determine baseline respiratory assessment (i.e., RR, skin color, respiratory effort, breath sounds, oxygen saturation).
5. Have child sit upright if possible as this will promote maximum lung expansion.
6. Pour medication into nebulizer cap and cover.
7. Fasten T-piece to top of cap. This provides the connector for the mouthpiece.
8. Fasten mouthpiece and mask to end of T-piece. The other end of the T-piece should have a short length of tubing.
9. Attach tubing to bottom of nebulizer cup and attach other end of tubing to air compressor.
10. Adjust wall oxygen valve to 6 liters/minute or less.
11. Child should breath slowly and deeply through mouthpiece and mask until medication has been nebulized (should take about 10 minutes).
12. Reassess respiratory status and client response to procedure (i.e., RR, skin color, respiratory effort, breath sounds, oxygen saturation).

URINARY CATHETERIZATION

NIC Intervention Label and Definition (0580): Urinary Catheterization—Insertion of a Catheter into the Bladder for Temporary or Permanent Drainage of Urine

NIC Intervention Label and Definition (0582): Urinary Catheterization Intermittent—Regular Periodic Use of a Catheter to Empty the Bladder

NIC Intervention Label and Definition (1876): Tube Care Urinary—Management of a Patient with Urinary Drainage Equipment

A urinary catheter is a rubber or plastic device used to drain urine from the bladder. A physician's order is necessary for this procedure. Intermittent catheterization may be used to obtain a urine sample or to relieve bladder distension. Indwelling catheters are left in place to keep the bladder empty, prevent retention, or to accurately measure urine output. In the acute care setting, the procedure is performed under strict sterile technique.

SIZE AND TYPE OF URINE CATHETERS

Child's Weight	Size and Type of Catheter
<3 kg	5 French feeding tube or straight catheter
3–8 kg	5–8 French straight or indwelling catheter
8–11 kg	8–10 French straight or indwelling catheter
11–14 kg	10 French straight or indwelling catheter
14–24 kg	10–12 French straight or indwelling catheter
24–32 kg	12 French straight or indwelling catheter

Procedure:

1. Gather necessary equipment: catheter, urethral catheterization tray, sterile gloves, Betadine swab sticks (or cleansing solution specified by agency), sterile lubricant (water soluble), 10-cc sterile syringe, sterile water, closed drainage bag (indwelling catherization only), tape.
2. Wash hands.
3. Prepare the child and family for the procedure in order to enhance co-operation and reduce anxiety or fear. Remember to provide for utmost privacy. Be sure to obtain adequate lighting.
4. Place child in recumbent position. It is helpful to have disposable pad underneath child in case of soiling from povidone-iodine.
5. Prepare sterile field. Open catheterization tray and drop sterile supplies on field.
6. Don sterile gloves.
7. Unfold waterproof underpad and place underneath child's buttocks.
8. Prepare cleansing solution and cotton balls. Some catheterization kits have prepared cleansing swabs.
9. Open sterile water-soluble lubricant.
10. Check catheter balloon by inflating and deflating it with sterile water.
11. Cleanse area properly.
    a. Female: separate labia with nondominant hand; cleanse labia and meatus from posterior to anterior using each swab only once
    b. Male: hold penis shaft with nondominant hand; cleanse meatus and clean outward in circular motion using each swab only once
12. Insert catheter.
    a. Female: hold catheter in sterile hand; lubricate tip of catheter; insert downward into urinary meatus; insert to hub and inflate balloon with recommended amount of sterile water.
    b. Male: hold catheter in sterile hand; lubricate tip; hold shaft of penis perpendicular to the body; insert catheter into urinary meatus

slowly and gently (never insert catheter when there is an erection); insert to hub and inflate balloon with recommended amount of sterile water.

13. Connect catheter to closed urinary collection bag. Attach drainage bag to bed below level of bladder and secure with tape (outer thigh for male, inner thigh for female).

CHAPTER 6

COMMON HEALTH PROBLEMS

ACUTE GLOMERULONEPHRITIS (AGN)
Brief Description

AGN is a disorder in which immune complexes deposit along the glomerular membrane. Most cases follow streptococcal, pneumococcal, or viral infections. There is a latent period of 10–21 days between infection and the onset of symptoms. Glomerular capillary loops become swollen and infiltrated, causing decreased filtration of plasma. This noninfectious renal disorder primarily affects school-age children. Recovery is spontaneous and children generally recover completely.

History and Physical Assessment Findings

Laboratory findings include increased BUN and creatinine, positive anti-streptolysin O (ASO) titre, and reduced serum complement (C3) activity. Urine is smoke colored, tea colored, or grossly bloody. Proteinuria is present. Patients commonly report a history of strep throat or other infection 2 weeks before symptoms. Urine output is decreased. Child has edema (especially facial and periorbital). Physical examination findings (e.g., edema, increased blood pressure [BP], increased weight) vary depending on level of renal involvement. Manifestations range from minimal to severe. Edematous phase can last up to 3 weeks with child feeling apathetic during that time. Increasing urine output and decreasing weight indicate improvement.

Nursing Care

Supportive nursing care is indicated. Children with mild cases (normal BP and urine output) are treated as outpatients. Close assessment of vital signs, weight, and intake and output are essential. Child may be placed on fluid and sodium restrictions if urine output is significantly low. Antihypertensive medications may be indicated. Antibiotics are prescribed if child has persistent streptococcal infection.

Related Nursing Diagnoses	NOC Outcomes	NIC Interventions
• *Excess fluid volume*	• Electrolyte and acid-base balance • Fluid balance • Hydration	• Fluid management • Fluid monitoring • Hypervolemic management
• *Disturbed body image*	• Body image	• Body image enhancement • Coping enhancement
• *Fatigue*	• Activity tolerance • Energy conservation	• Energy management • Nutrition management

AGGRESSIVENESS

Brief Description

Children with *aggressiveness* exhibit behavior in which they attempt to hurt another person or destroy another's property. Often the behavior is unprovoked and is exhibited through physical attacks, destruction of property, extreme impulsivity, and noncompliance. Frustration, modeling another's behavior, and reinforcement seem to increase aggressive behavior. This behavioral problem is influenced by biologic, sociocultural, and familial variables.

History and Physical Assessment Findings

History of hostility, combativeness, and fighting is common. Majority have associated social impairments, psychiatric disorders, or adult criminal behavior.

Nursing Care

Treatment includes caregiver management training, teaching child new coping skills, family therapy, and psychopharmacologic intervention. Early intervention is the goal. Referral to psychiatrist or psychologist is often necessary.

Related Nursing Diagnoses	NOC Outcomes	NIC Interventions
• *Injury, risk for*	• Risk control • Safety behavior: personal	• Behavior modification • Parent education • Patient contracting • Self-modification assistance • Surveillance: safety *(Continued)*

Related Nursing Diagnoses	NOC Outcomes	NIC Interventions
• *Violence: other-directed, risk for*	• Aggression control • Impulse control	• Anger control assistance • Environmental management: violence prevention • Impulse control training
• *Social isolation*	• Social interaction skills • Social involvement	• Behavior modification: social skills • Self-awareness enhancement • Socialization enhancement
• *Interrupted family processes*	• Family coping • Family functioning	• Family integration promotion • Family process maintenance • Family support

ANXIETY

Brief Description

Children with *anxiety* have general uneasiness and apprehension. Anxiety is different from fear; fears are more specific in nature and generally are limited problems that disappear with growth. Anxiety usually manifests as a panic attack. Panic attacks are unexpected events.

History and Physical Assessment
Findings

Panic attacks are associated with at least four of the following symptoms: shortness of breath (SOB), dizziness or faintness, palpitations or tachycardia, shakiness, sweating, feeling of choking, nausea or abdominal discomfort, numbness or tingling, flushing, chest pain or discomfort, fear of dying, and fear of losing control.

Nursing Care

Therapy with a mental health professional is indicated for children with anxiety. Psychopharmacologic treatment has not proven effective in children with anxiety disorders.

Related Nursing Diagnoses	NOC Outcomes	NIC Interventions
• *Anxiety*	• Anxiety control	• Anxiety reduction
• *Ineffective coping*	• Coping	• Coping enhancement • Support group
• *Disturbed sleep pattern*	• Anxiety control	• Coping enhancement • Sleep enhancement

APPENDICITIS

Brief Description

Appendicitis is the most common cause of abdominal surgery in the pediatric population. It is caused by obstruction of the lumen of the appendix (usually from fecalith). Obstruction causes compression of blood vessels and ischemia. Early recognition is essential in order to prevent perforation and resulting peritonitis.

History and Physical Assessment Findings

Abdominal pain is a common finding. Generally, pain begins as diffuse and cramping in periumbilical area and then increases in severity while migrating to right lower quadrant (McBurney's point). Associated nausea, vomiting, and anorexia are common complaints. Low grade fever is present early in the disease and can significantly rise if there is perforation and peritonitis. Rebound tenderness, decreased or absent bowel sounds, constipation, difficulty ambulating, and irritability are other signs or symptoms. Laboratory studies include CBC and C-reactive protein. Diagnostic studies include ultrasonography and CT scan. Because many abdominal infectious and inflammatory conditions present similarly, diagnosis is not straightforward.

Nursing Care

Accurate history and pain assessment are essential interventions. Treatment includes IV hydration, IV antibiotic administration, and surgical removal (appendectomy). For non-perforated appendicitis, laparoscopic surgical techniques are available. Postoperative care involves pain assessment, pain control, prevention and monitoring of abdominal distension, hydration, antibiotic administration, wound care, and psychosocial support. Postoperative care is prolonged if there is perforation.

Related Nursing Diagnoses	NOC Outcomes	NIC Interventions
• *Acute pain*	• Comfort level • Pain control • Pain level	• Medication management • Pain management *(Continued)*

Related Nursing Diagnoses	NOC Outcomes	NIC Interventions
		• Patient-controlled analgesia assistance • Positioning
• *Risk for infection*	• Infection status • Wound healing: primary intention	• Infection protection • Incision site care • Vital signs monitoring • Teaching: procedure and treatment
• *Interrupted family processes*	• Family coping	• Coping enhancement

ASTHMA (REACTIVE AIRWAY DISEASE)
Brief Description

Asthma is a chronic inflammatory pulmonary disease that results from a wide range of stimuli (e.g., pollen, dust, viruses, smoke, strong odors, roach dander, animals). It is the most common chronic disease in children, and results in increased irritability of tracheobronchial tree with airway obstruction of varying degrees. Asthma episode may or may not be reversible following therapy or spontaneously. Children are more vulnerable to airway obstruction because of their small airway and compromised collateral ventilation. Narrowing of airway caused by smooth muscle contraction of airway (bronchospasm), edema and inflammation of tracheobronchial mucosa, and excessive secretion of submucosal glands, which causes mucous plugging. Exacerbations are characterized as recurrent episodes of wheezing, increased work of breathing (WOB), cough, and chest tightness.

Classification of Asthma Severity
Step 1: Mild Intermittent Asthma

Symptoms ≤2x/wk

Asymptomatic with normal peak expiratory flow (PEF) between exacerbations

Exacerbations brief (from few hours to few days) with varying intensity

Nighttime symptoms ≤2x/mo

Forced expiratory volume over 1 min (FEV_1)/PEF ≥80% of predicted value, with variability <20%

Step 2: Mild Persistent Asthma

Symptoms >2x/wk but <1x/day

Exacerbations may affect activity

Nighttime symptoms >2x/mo

FEV_1/PEF 80% of predicted value with variability of 20%–30%

Step 3: Moderate Persistent Asthma

Daily symptoms
Daily use of inhaled, short-acting β_2-agonist
Exacerbations affect activity
Exacerbations $\geq$2x/wk; may last for days
Nighttime symptoms >1x/wk
FEV_1/PEF between 60% and 80% of predicted value with 30% variability

Step 4: Severe Persistent Asthma

Continual symptoms
Limited physical activity
Frequent exacerbations
Frequent nighttime symptoms
FEV_1/PEF <60% of predicted value with >30% variability (Kemper, 1997)

Diagnostic Tests

The following tests need to be performed:

- Complete blood cell count (CBC)—leukocytosis occasionally found, eosinophilia frequently found
- Serum immunoglobulin E (IgE)
- Pulmonary function tests
- PEF
- Chest X ray
- Allergy testing

History and Physical Assessment Findings

Obtain thorough history including medications routinely used at home. Children with asthma often have a history of eczema, recurrent bronchitis, and persistent cough. Symptoms are usually worse at night. Assess exposure to triggers, especially environmental tobacco smoke (ETS). Respiratory assessment should include respiratory rate, presence of dyspnea, retractions, nasal flaring, and use of accessory muscles. Skin color and capillary refill time should be noted. Lungs should be auscultated for unequal breath sounds, crackles, or wheezes. Cardiac rate and rhythm should be assessed, especially during drug therapy.

Nursing Care

Assess child's and caregiver's understanding of disease process and use of medications to manage. Provide client teaching related to avoidance of allergens or triggers. Administer drug therapy and teach caregivers and child what drugs do to help asthma and whether they are short- or long-term use drugs. Short-acting β_2-agonists such as albuterol may be used PO or by inhalation. Cromolyn and inhaled steroids are long-acting, preventive drugs. Steroids are also given PO or IV for acute exacerbations. Provide oxygen p.r.n. and monitor pulse oximeter readings. Place in Fowler's or semi-Fowler's position to facilitate breathing. Provide teaching related to home care including use of PEF meter and how to manage asthma according to PEF reading. Children >6 year can be taught to use a PEF meter; all children discharged with diagnosis of asthma should have a written management plan that is reviewed with caregiver and child and a copy sent home with them.

Related Nursing Diagnoses	NOC Outcomes	NIC Interventions
• *Suffocation, risk for*	• Respiratory status: ventilation • Risk control • Safety behavior: home physical environment	• Airway management • Environmental management: safety • Respiratory monitoring
• *Airway clearance, ineffective*	• Respiratory status: airway patency • Respiratory status: gas exchange • Respiratory status: ventilation	• Acid-base monitoring • Airway management • Oxygen therapy • Positioning • Respiratory monitoring • Ventilation assistance
• *Activity intolerance*	• Activity tolerance • Endurance	• Activity therapy • Energy management
• *Interrupted family processes*	• Family coping • Family environment: internal	• Coping enhancement • Family integration promotion • Family process maintenance • Normalization promotion • Parent education
• *Health maintenance, ineffective*	• Health seeking behavior • Knowledge: health behaviors • Knowledge: treatment regimen	• Health education • Risk identification • Teaching: disease process • Teaching: procedure/ treatment

ATTENTION DEFICIT HYPERACTIVITY DISORDER (ADHD)

Brief Description

ADHD is a chronic neurobehavioral disorder that can interfere with a child's ability to inhibit behavior, function effectively in goal-oriented activities, or regulate activity level in developmentally appropriate ways. Three behavioral subtypes are defined by the American Psychiatric Association *Diagnostic and Statistical Manual of Mental Disorders, 4th Edition* (*DSM-IV*). Subtypes are predominately inattentive, predominately hyperactive or impulsive, and combined. Symptoms must be present before the age of 7 and persist for greater than 6 months for this diagnosis to be made. Some children can be diagnosed earlier, but rarely before age 4 years for accurate diagnosis. The underlying problem is still unclear; however, there are many theories. One is that the affected child cannot produce enough norepinephrine, a neurochemical transmitter, to allow messages to be transmitted effectively from one neuron to another to complete the transmission.

History and Physical Assessment Findings

Disorder usually affects all aspects of child's life but is most pervasive in school-related activities. No specific diagnostic measures are currently available. Diagnosis is based on evaluation of child's behavior in multiple settings, such as school, home, and day care, by multiple people having contact with the child. A plethora of behavioral checklists is available to aid caregivers, teachers, and school nurses in assessing behavioral characteristics. Initial assessment should include questions about chronic problems, behavioral problems, how child is managed at home (e.g., behavior modification), routines, and medications and times of administration. Also assess when medication seems to be wearing off and how long it lasts in the current setting. Ritalin (usually first drug used) lasts 3–5 hours.

Nursing Care

Provide a safe environment, try as much as possible to maintain routines as they are at home, and ensure provision of medication at a time most appropriate for the child's care. Stimulant-type medications are best taken in the morning to maximize effectiveness and minimize side effects. Communicate to family and all caregivers that child has a behavior problem that has multiple origins including an underlying central nervous system (CNS) basis and needs understanding, reassurance, and routine in a new setting. Encourage family involvement in plan and care.

Related Nursing Diagnoses	NOC Outcomes	NIC Interventions
• *Self-esteem, chronic low, potential for*	• Self-esteem • Depression level • Quality of life	• Self-esteem enhancement • Mood management
• *Social interaction, impaired*	• Child development • Social interaction skills • Social involvement	• Behavior modification: social skills • Developmental enhancement • Socialization enhancement
• *Interrupted family processes*	• Family coping • Family functioning • Parenting	• Family integrity promotion • Coping enhancement • Family process maintenance • Normalization promotion • Parenting promotion

AUTISM
Brief Description

Autism is a complex developmental syndrome involving impaired brain functioning, intellectual deficits, and behavioral deficits. Children with autism demonstrate bizarre social interactions, communication, and behavior. Generally manifests in children ages 18–36 months. More commonly found in males. Autism is usually severely disabling. Autism has an unknown etiology. Current evidence suggests multiple biologic causes. Immunization with measles-mumps-rubella (MMR) vaccine does not appear to be a cause of autism.

History and Physical Assessment Findings

Abnormal electroencephalogram (EEG), seizures, delayed development of hand dominance, persistent primitive reflexes, elevated blood serotonin, and cerebellar vermal hypoplasia are common findings. Classic sign is inability to maintain eye contact with another person. Language and speech delays are common in children with autism. Majority have some degree of mental retardation.

Nursing Care

Most children require lifelong adult supervision. No cure for this syndrome exists. Children with autism need highly structured and intensive behavioral modification programs; these have shown to be most effective therapy. Goal of care is to promote positive reinforcement, increase social awareness, develop communication skills, and decrease unacceptable behaviors. Providing structured environment is a critical aspect of care. During child's hospitalization, caregivers are essential to care planning and should remain with child as much as possible. Physical contact should be avoided because it is distressing to children with autism.

Related Nursing Diagnoses	NOC Outcomes	NIC Interventions
• *Social interaction, impaired*	• Child development • Social interaction skills • Social involvement	• Complex relationship building • Developmental enhancement • Socialization enhancement
• *Communication: verbal, impaired*	• Communication ability • Communication: expressive ability • Communication: receptive ability	• Communication enhancement
• *Caregiver role strain, risk for*	• Family coping • Family functioning • Knowledge: health resources • Rest	• Caregiver support • Coping enhancement • Emotional support • Parenting promotion • Respite care
• *Growth and development, delayed*	• Child development	• Developmental care • Developmental enhancement
• *Self-mutilation, risk for*	• Self-mutilation restraint	• Behavior management: self-harm • Environmental management, safety

BRONCHIOLITIS
Brief Description
Bronchiolitis is an acute viral infection of the small airways in the lower respiratory tract causing airway hypersensitivity, edema, and inflammation. Majority of cases result from respiratory syncytial virus (RSV). Other viruses such as parainfluenza virus and adenoviruses can also cause bronchiolitis. Rate of infection peaks in months between November and March; average age of those affected is 2–9 months. Bronchiolitis is one of the most common

causes of pediatric hospitalization, although most children with this illness are managed at home. This infection may be life-threatening especially in young infants and children with cardiac and respiratory disease history (e.g., congenital heart disease, bronchopulmonary dysplasia).

History and Physical Assessment Findings

Usually involves a history of recent upper respiratory infection with symptoms of cough, nasal stuffiness, and fever. As illness progresses, symptoms become more severe and result in increased work of breathing. Usually include an increased respiratory rate, shallow respiratory pattern, nasal flaring, retractions, and tachycardia. Children with severe illness may exhibit decreased air entry and lethargy. Diagnosis made on basis of the history, physical examination, chest X ray (shows hyperinflation or inflammation), and positive viral culture (nasopharyngeal swab or wash).

Nursing Care

Ongoing close assessment is necessary. Because of the structure of the child's airway, deteriorating changes can occur very rapidly. Treatment is generally supportive in nature. Oxygen and respiratory therapies are often ordered. O_2 mist tent may be used. Continuous pulse oximetry is indicated, especially early in illness. Interventions aimed at keeping airway clear should be implemented (e.g., suctioning, increasing height of head of bed). Nebulized albuterol or racemic epinephrine may be used to treat some children with bronchiolitis. Steroids and antibiotics are generally not helpful. Use of ribavirin (via small-particle aerosol) is usually reserved for those with severe symptoms and those with preexisting cardiopulmonary states. Because of teratogenic effects of ribavirin, pregnant health care workers should not provide care for children receiving ribavirin therapy. The American Academy of Pediatrics (AAP) recommends that children with a history of chronic lung disease or those born prior to 32 weeks' gestation be given Palivizumab or RSV immune globulin (RSV-IGIV) as prophylaxis to prevent RSV infection.

Related Nursing Diagnoses	NOC Outcomes	NIC Interventions
• *Breathing pattern, ineffective*	• Respiratory status: airway patency • Respiratory status: ventilation • Vital signs status	• Airway management • Airway suctioning • Respiratory monitoring • Ventilation assistance • Vital signs monitoring *(Continued)*

• *Gas exchange, impaired*	• Electrolyte and acid-base balance • Respiratory status: gas exchange • Respiratory status: ventilation • Tissue perfusion: pulmonary • Vital signs status	• Acid-base management • Airway management • Laboratory data interpretation • Oxygen therapy • Respiratory monitoring • Ventilation assistance • Vital signs monitoring
• *Fluid volume, deficient, risk for*	• Fluid balance • Hydration • Nutritional status: food and fluid intake • Electrolyte and acid-base balance	• Fluid/electrolyte management • Fluid monitoring • Hypovolemic management • Intravenous therapy
• *Knowledge, deficient*	• Knowledge	• Teaching: disease process • Teaching: procedure and treatment

CANCER
Brief Description
Cause of *cancer* in children is unknown, but genetic alterations resulting in unregulated proliferation of cells, genetic inheritance, chromosomal abnormalities, immune system suppression, Epstein-Barr virus, environmental agents, power line exposure, and certain drugs all have been proposed as possible causative factors in various types of cancers in children.

Presenting Signs and Symptoms
Fever
Pain
Limping
Anemia
Bruising or petechiae
Infection
Fatigue
Painless abdominal mass
Weight loss
Palpable lymph nodes
Behavioral changes
Night sweats
Seizure activity

    Neurologic changes
    Leukocoria (white reflection in pupil)
    Early morning headaches

Diagnostic Work-Up

    History and physical examination
    Laboratory studies
    Bone marrow aspiration
    Diagnostic imaging
    Surgical staging, biopsy

Treatment Modalities

Child usually placed on a protocol involving any or all of the following:
    Surgery
    Chemotherapy
    Radiation
    Bone marrow transplant

Common Types of Cancer in Children

Leukemia

Leukemia is a group of malignant disorders of the bone marrow and lymphatic system and is the most common form of childhood cancer. Two forms recognized in children are *acute lymphoid leukemia* (ALL), which is the most common, and *acute myelogenous leukemia* (AML).

Lymphoma

Lymphoma is a group of neoplastic diseases that arise from the lymphoid and hemopoietic systems and are divided into Hodgkin's and non-Hodgkin's lymphoma (NHL). Both have four stages depending on tumor spread and lymph node involvement.

Brain Tumors

Brain tumors are the most common solid tumors in children and include the following types:

- Low- or high-grade astrocytoma—Most common pediatric brain tumor that infiltrates the brain parenchyma without distinct boundaries
- Medulloblastoma (primitive neuroectodermal tumor [PNET])—Fast growing, highly malignant
- Cerebellar astrocytoma—Slow growing if low grade

- Brainstem glioma— Often grows very large before causes symptoms; most are highly resistant to therapy
- Ependymoma—Most invade the ventricles, obstructing cerebrospinal fluid (CSF) flow

Neuroblastoma

In *neuroblastoma*, tumors arise from embryonic neural crest cells, so majority of tumors come from the adrenal gland or from the retroperitoneal sympathetic chain. Most common primary site is the abdomen. Also has staging system based on tumor dissemination.

Bone Tumors

There are two types of *bone tumors:*

- Osteogenic sarcoma—Most common type of bone tumor in children that arises from the osseous tissue. More than half occur in the femur, especially the distal part, with the rest involving the humerus, tibia, pelvis, jaw, and phalanges.
- Ewing's sarcoma (PNET of the bone)—Arises in the marrow spaces of the bone.

Other Solid Tumors

- Wilms' tumor (nephroblastoma)—Tumor of the kidney; has hereditary component. Most common intraabdominal tumor of children.
- Rhabdomyosarcoma—Most common soft-tissue tumor in children; arises in striated muscle. Most common sites are head and neck, especially the orbit.
- Retinoblastoma—Malignant tumor; arises from retina. Can be inherited.

Side Effects of Treatment

Infection	Hemorrhagic cystitis
Hemorrhage	Alopecia
Anemia	Nausea and vomiting
Altered nutrition	Mucosal ulceration
Neurologic problems	Lowered body defenses

Nursing Care

Prepare client and family for diagnostic and treatment procedures. Involve play therapy as appropriate. Provide support for family during diagnostic and treatment processes by answering questions; encouraging verbalization of fears and concerns; and involving social services, chaplains, and support groups as appropriate. Administer chemotherapy as ordered and monitor for side effects of all medications. Protect from infection and administer antiemetics before and p.r.n. after chemotherapy to prevent and treat nausea and vomiting. Assess for pain and administer analgesics as ordered; implement pain management techniques. Ensure adequate nutrition by encouraging intake of small portions of anything tolerated by the child. Provide meticulous skin care, including oral mucous membranes, to help prevent breakdown. Encourage developmentally appropriate activities. Provide education about disease process and needed care as well as for home care as appropriate.

Related Nursing Diagnoses	NOC Outcomes	NIC Interventions
• *Injury, risk for*	• Immune status • Risk control	• Surveillance: safety • Health screening
• *Risk for infection*	• Immune status • Infection status • Knowledge: infection control • Wound healing	• Infection control • Infection protection • Incision site care • Wound care
• *Fluid volume deficient, risk for*	• Fluid balance • Hydration • Nutritional status: food and fluid intake • Electrolyte and acid-base balance	• Fluid and electrolyte management • Fluid monitoring • Intravenous therapy • Nutrition management • Nutrition monitoring
• *Oral mucous membrane, impaired*	• Oral health • Tissue integrity: skin and mucous membranes	• Oral health restoration
• *Nutrition, imbalanced: less than body requirements*	• Nutritional status • Nutritional status: food and fluid intake	• Nutrition monitoring • Nutrition management • Weight gain assistance
• *Skin integrity, risk for impaired*	• Tissue integrity: skin and mucous membranes • Wound healing	• Skin surveillance • Wound care • Incision site care
• *Disturbed body image*	• Body image • Child development • Grief resolution • Psychosocial adjustment: life change	• Anticipatory guidance • Body image enhancement • Coping enhancement • Developmental enhancement

(Continued)

	• Self-esteem	• Grief work facilitation • Self-esteem enhancement
• *Acute pain*	• Comfort level • Pain control • Pain: disruptive effects • Pain level	• Analgesic administration • Conscious sedation • Medication management • Pain management • Patient-controlled analgesic (PCA) assistance
• *Pain, chronic*	• Comfort level • Pain control • Pain: disruptive effects • Pain level • Pain: psychological response	• Analgesic administration • Behavior modification • Coping enhancement • Medication management • Mood management • Pain management • Patient contracting • Patient-controlled analgesia (PCA) assistance
• *Fear*	• Anxiety control • Fear control	• Anxiety reduction • Coping enhancement • Security enhancement
• *Interrupted family processes*	• Family coping • Family functioning • Family health status • Parenting	• Coping enhancement • Family integrity promotion • Family process maintenance • Family support • Normalization promotion • Parent education
• *Grieving, anticipatory*	• Coping • Grief resolution • Psychosocial adjustment: life change	• Anticipatory guidance • Coping enhancement • Grief work facilitation • Family support

CARE OF THE CHILD AND FAMILY WITH CHRONIC ILLNESS

The number of children with chronic diseases and conditions are increasing. These children and their families have unique responses, needs, and nursing care requirements.

Effect on Child

The impact of chronic illness on a child is influenced by age of onset. Unpredictability can lead to frequent hospitalizations and appointments with health care practitioners that interrupt normalcy. May have associated pain and discomfort. Child may have misinformation or not enough information and fear the unknown. Growth and development may be restricted, which makes these children different from their peers. They may be unable to participate in normal activities, which also makes them feel different from their peers. May have decreased feelings of worth and feel guilty for daily care requirements.

Child's Response

Child may respond by being angry, uncooperative, and belligerent. May show signs of depression, resignation, or confusion. May also feel isolated and withdrawn, although some children seem to rise to each new challenge and adapt quite well.

Effect on Family

Family will grieve for loss of normal child and his or her potential and feel a strain on all relationships, stress over daily care requirements and financial burden, loss of control, and isolation.

Caregiver's Response

Type of chronic illness and amount of positive feedback from child affect caregiver's response. Caregivers may go through denial, grief, guilt, anger, helplessness, fear, and loneliness. These feelings may potentiate at every missed milestone, such as first steps, first day at school, or getting a driver's license.

Sibling's Response

Sibling may feel forgotten and less important than and jealous of sick sibling. May get angry and resent caregivers being away all the time. May feel guilty, sad, isolated, or lonely, and may act out to get attention.

Nursing Intervention

General

Use primary nurse as much as possible and admit to same unit in hospital each admission. Use developmental approach instead of one based on age to help emphasize abilities and not disabilities. Focus on strengths. Encourage normalcy as much as is realistic. As families learn about their child and his or her condition, they become experts for that child and need to be recognized as such.

Child

Depends on developmental level and condition. Assess child's understanding of illness and how he or she is responding and adapting. Provide support for coping and allow and encourage expression of feelings. Promote normal growth and development. Prepare for changes and treatments. Encourage participation in and responsibility for care and control as much as possible. Encourage peer and sibling support and help with care; help them understand expectations and responsibilities. Focus on abilities. Encourage association with peers with same problems if possible, and encourage involvement in decision making.

Caregivers

Assess how well caregivers are adapting to the child's illness. Determine and provide knowledge, skills, and resources needed to help them adapt. Provide information on normal growth and development so they can encourage development of their child. Encourage involvement of all caregivers. Clarify needs of each caregiver; they may be in different stages of adapting because of different amounts of contact with child and health care system. Encourage normalization and realistic expectations of child and of family functioning. Encourage open communication. Allow verbalization of frustrations and feelings, and respond in a caring, nonjudgmental, nondefensive manner. Help caregivers get involved in support groups if appropriate and help them set up their own support systems.

Siblings

Encourage visitation and involvement in care during hospitalization if appropriate for sibling's age and child's condition. Assess sibling's understanding of child's illness and his or her adjustment to it. Provide supportive communication. Encourage phone calls to caregivers and sick child. Give positive strokes when present and recognize sibling's presence and feelings.

CARING FOR THE DYING CHILD AND THE FAMILY

Death is a difficult nursing situation because it causes nurses to examine their feelings about death—their own and others. Working with dying children and their families can be both challenging and rewarding. To be most effective, nurses need to be aware of how different age groups conceptualize and react to death—their own and others.

Perceptions by Age Groups

Infants or Toddlers

Concept:	None
Reaction to own impending:	Take cues from loved ones' responses
Reaction to death of others:	React to the separation and loss of consistency by regressing, becoming irritable, and developing sleeping and eating problems.

Preschoolers (3–5 years)

Concept:	Is separation; temporary, gradual, and reversible
Reaction to own impending:	Is punishment for bad thoughts or actions
Reaction to death of others:	May feel guilty, as if their thoughts or actions were responsible; may regress or show denial with inappropriate behavior

School-Age Children (6–11 years)

Concept:	Is not reversible but also is not inevitable; may see it as destructive or look for natural or physical explanations
Reaction to own impending:	May show fear of the unknown; need help to maintain control of own body. May be verbally uncooperative because of fear; show "flight or fight" reaction
Reaction to death of others:	Feel guilt and responsibility; ask many questions to help arrange facts into concrete and logical understanding

Adolescents (12–18 years)

Concept: Is irreversible, universal, and inevitable. Is a personal but far-off event. Explain it physiologically and theologically.

Reaction to own
impending: Reject death because it interferes with their establishment of identity. Become alienated from their peers and unable to talk to caregivers. Use denial and rationalization. Are present oriented and worry about physical changes that may further alienate them from their peers.

Reaction to death
of others: Feel guilt and shame. This group has more difficulty coping with death than do the other age groups and may be unable to accept support.

Caregiver Responses

Initial (When informed of life-threatening illness or condition of child)

Shock, disbelief
Anger
Overprotectiveness
Anxiety
Ambivalence

After the Loss

Shock, confusion, decreased sense of reality
Guilt, anger
Sorrow
Depression
Loneliness, yearning
Helplessness, despair, fear
Reorganization, reconciliation, relief

Caregivers may be in different stages of acceptance and may respond differently. Caregivers may have reached acceptance before nurse does. May be reconciled to death of child long before child dies. Child's death after lengthy, painful illness may be a relief. Need to be helped to understand that this is alright and should not feel guilty for their feelings.

Sibling Responses

Siblings respond according to their age group and developmental stage. Reaction also depends on caregivers' reactions, amount of time they have had to adjust, and amount of involvement and inclusion they have had. Often feel isolated and guilty. May also feel that they are not as important as child who died and that they need to replace that child and be strong, be good, and not talk about their sibling. May have been sheltered and left out.

Nursing Care

Nurses may need help dealing with their own feelings before they are able to help the dying child and his or her family. Seek assistance from experienced nurses, social worker, or chaplain. All nurses are initially uncomfortable because it forces us to face our children's and our own mortality. Be careful to not impose your own views, values, or explanations on the family.

Child

The dying child needs accurate, honest information and time to think it out. Process needs to be gradual with increasingly open communication between child, caregivers, and nurse. When child asks questions, ask what he or she thinks is happening to find out what he or she understands, how he or she feels, and what child really wants to know. Be sure to discuss with caregivers beforehand about how they want to handle communication and what they want child to know. Even though open communication is best, it is still the caregivers' right to determine what they feel is best for the child. Help correct any misinformation.

Family

Assess resources and ability to cope; intervene and refer as necessary. Caregivers also need honest and complete information to empower them to make appropriate choices. They need information on how to tell the child, siblings, and other family members. They need an opportunity to express their feelings in a supportive environment. Respect their wishes in regard to what they want child to know, but help them realize that trust fosters trust. After the death of the child, stay with the family or have a chaplain or social worker available. Ensure the child's dignity. Encourage expression of memories and feelings. Answer questions honestly. Allow them to stay with the child as long as they wish. Give them time and privacy to say goodbye. Help with arrangements, ensure closure, and encourage current ties with nursing staff.

CELIAC DISEASE

Brief Description

Celiac disease is a chronic, genetic malabsorption disorder. It is more common in children of White European descent. The disease is characterized by intolerance for gluten, which is a protein found in wheat, oats, barley, and rye. An inability to digest glutenin causes an accumulation of glutamine, an amino acid that is toxic to intestinal mucosal cells. Absorption is impaired as a result of damage to the villi within the small intestine.

History and Physical Assessment Findings

Symptoms of Celiac disease usually appear once solid foods have been introduced into the diet. The classic signs and symptoms are diarrhea, failure to thrive, and abdominal pain. Additional symptoms include vomiting, anemia, and irritability. Muscle wasting, abdominal distension, and delayed dentition are often seen with delayed diagnosis. Additionally, undiagnosed cases may lead to malignancies such as lymphoma and carcinoma. Celiac disease is diagnosed through fecal fat analysis, duodenal biopsy, and signs of improvement when gluten products are withdrawn from the diet.

Nursing Care

Patient teaching regarding a lifetime gluten-free diet is required. Assessments of growth and developmental milestones should be done.

Related Nursing Diagnoses	NOC Outcomes	NIC Interventions
• *Nutrition, imbalanced: less than body requirements*	• Nutritional status	• Nutrition management
• *Risk for delayed growth and development*	• Growth • Physical maturation	• Nutrition therapy
• *Knowledge deficient (parental and child)*	• Knowledge: disease process	• Teaching: disease process

CENTRAL NERVOUS SYSTEM INFECTIONS

Brief Description

CNS infections include bacterial meningitis, aseptic or viral meningitis, encephalitis, and brain abscess. Both bacterial and viral meningitis result in inflammation of the meninges. Bacterial meningitis is more serious than viral meningitis and is sometimes fatal. Encephalitis is inflammation of the brain; often the meninges are also inflamed. Common pathogens associated with bacterial meningitis include *Haemophilus influenzae, Streptococcus pneumoniae, Neisseria meningitides,* group B streptococcus, *Staphylococcus aureus,* and pseudomonas. Aseptic meningitis is most commonly caused by enterovirus. Encephalitis usually follows other infections such as measles, varicella, mumps, herpes, Epstein-Barr infection, and influenza. Common pathogens associated with brain abscesses include *S. aureus,* group A streptococcus, *H. influenza,* gram-negative enteric bacteria, and fungi.

History and Physical Assessment Findings

Children with CNS infections may have a history of immune compromise, travel outside of country, lack of immunization, and vector exposure (e.g., mosquito). They generally exhibit signs and symptoms such as nuchal rigidity, headache, behavior changes, seizures, photophobia, cranial nerve alterations, and fever. Positive Kernig's or Brudzinski sign may be present. Depending on the causative factor, children may also exhibit other signs such as rash (petechiae or purpura), vomiting, and diarrhea. CSF examination (lumbar puncture) yields organisms and alterations in cell count, protein, and glucose. Blood and urine cultures may also be positive. CBC results demonstrate increase in white blood cells (WBCs).

Nursing Care

Initial care is considered an emergency. Careful assessment of neurologic status is required. Child is placed in isolation, and standard precautions and droplet precautions are used until pathogen is identified. First priority of care for children with bacterial CNS infections is to administer IV antibiotics. Doses may be required for up to 3 weeks depending on organism and virulence. Corticosteroids (e.g., dexamethasone), anticonvulsants, and antipyretics often given. Important to administer steroids before or with first dose of antibiotics. Antiviral (e.g., acyclovir) may be prescribed for those with aseptic meningitis. Surgery or aspiration may be indicated in children with brain abscesses. Accurate measurement of intake and output necessary; child may be placed on fluid restriction to prevent cerebral edema, increased intracranial pressure (IP), and syndrome of inappropriate antidiuretic hormone secretion (SIADH). Reduction of environmental stimuli is recommended.

Related Nursing Diagnoses	NOC Outcomes	NIC Interventions
• *Infection*	• Infection status • Immune status • Knowledge: infection control	• Infection control • Infection protection
• *Hyperthermia*	• Thermoregulation	• Fever treatment • Temperature regulation • Vital signs monitoring
• *Tissue perfusion, ineffective*	• Neurological status: consciousness • Neurological status: central motor control • Tissue perfusion: cerebral	• Cerebral perfusion promotion • Intracranial pressure (ICP) monitoring • Neurologic monitoring
• *Sensory perception, disturbed*	• Cognitive orientation • Neurological status	• Neurological monitoring • Cognitive stimulation • Environmental management
• *Adaptive capacity: intracranial, decreased*	• Neurological status • Fluid balance	• Cerebral edema management • Cerebral perfusion promotion • Intracranial pressure (ICP) monitoring • Neurological monitoring
• *Coping: family, compromised*	• Caregiver emotional health • Caregiver-patient relationship • Caregiver stressors • Family coping • Family normalization	• Caregiver support • Coping enhancement • Emotional support • Family support • Normalization promotion

COMMUNICABLE DISEASES
Chickenpox (Varicella)

Infective Organism. Varicella-zoster virus (VZV) is a herpesvirus.

Sources. Humans.

Transmission. Direct contact with respiratory secretions; also airborne (droplet).

Incubation Period. Usually 14–16 days.

Period of communicability. Twenty-four hours before eruption of lesions (considered prodromal period) until after vesicles have crusted over (about day 6 or 7).

Signs and Symptoms. Pruritic rash begins on trunk as macules and progresses to vesicles and crusting. Child may have slight fever and decreased appetite.

Isolation. Airborne and contact precautions for ≥5 days after rash begins and for as long as rash is vesicular. For exposed susceptible clients, airborne and contact precautions for days 8–21 after onset in index client.

Nursing Care. Symptomatic. No aspirin because of increased risk of Reye's syndrome. Acetaminophen may delay crusting but can be used to control fever. Tepid bath with cornstarch may help with itching. Administer diphenhydramine hydrochloride (Benadryl) or hydroxyzine hydrochloride (Atarax) as ordered for itching. Keep child's nails short. Teach older child to push on itching lesions instead of scratching. Keep child cool to decrease itching and lesion formation. Sometimes treated with IV or PO acyclovir (IV for immunocompromised patients), but not recommended routinely for uncomplicated varicella in otherwise healthy child.

Complications. Local cellulitis from secondary infections, encephalitis, and Reye's syndrome.

Human Immunodeficiency Virus (HIV) Infection

Infective Organism. Human immunodeficiency virus type 1.

Sources. Humans.

Transmission. Predominant modes are via exposure to blood, semen, cervical secretions, and human milk from sexual contact; percutaneous or mucous membrane exposure, vertical from mother to infant at or around time of birth; and breastfeeding.

Incubation Period. Variable from months to years. Perinatally infected median age of onset is age 3 years. Those who acquire HIV other than perinatally usually develop serum antibodies to HIV within 6–12 weeks after infection.

Signs and Symptoms. Can present in any system. Most common manifestations include generalized lymphadenopathy, hepatomegaly and splenomegaly, failure to thrive, recurrent or persistent oral candidiasis, recurrent diarrhea, parotitis, cardiomyopathy, hepatitis, nephropathy, or CNS disease. Also may show developmental delay, lymphoid interstitial pneumonitis (LIP), recurrent invasive bacterial infections, and opportunistic infections such as *Pneumocystis carinii* pneumonia (PCP).

Diagnostic Testing.
- HIV enzyme-linked immunosorbent assay (ELISA)—Screening test for HIV antibody.
- HIV western blot—Confirmatory test used to check validity of ELISA test because western blot more precisely detects presence of antibodies to specific antigens.

The aforementioned tests are accurate in children >18 months.

- HIV p24 antigen assay—Tests for protein that surrounds the ribonucleic acid (RNA) and for reverse transcriptase of HIV.
- HIV deoxyribonucleic acid (DNA) polymerase chain reaction (PCR)— Standard current diagnostic test.
- HIV culture—HIV culture and HIV PCR are the most sensitive and specific tests to determine HIV infection in children who were perinatally exposed.

Classification. As of 1994 (Centers for Disease Control and Prevention [CDC], 1994), children with HIV infection are classified by three immunologic and three clinical categories.

Immunologic categories categorize by severity of immunosuppression caused by HIV infection. Age-specific CD4 counts and T-lymphocyte percentages determine category.

1. No evidence of suppression
2. Evidence of moderate suppression
3. Severe suppression

Clinical categories are used to provide a staging classification.

N. Not symptomatic
A. Mildly symptomatic
B. Moderately symptomatic
C. Severely symptomatic

The best prognosis is for a child classified as N1; poorest is C3. The CDC has established specific parameters and definitions. An E prefix means perinatally exposed.

Isolation. Universal blood and body fluid precautions.

Nursing Care. The goal of therapy for children with HIV infection is to slow the growth of the virus, while preventing and treating opportunistic infections. A variety of antiretroviral medications are used to interrupt the reproduction and function of viral particles. Guidelines for the use of antiretroviral agents are continually evolving. Many children have multiple hospitalizations and need the same care as other children with chronic or lifethreatening illnesses. You need to help support family and child emotionally by listening and helping set up services as needed. Use social services and all resources available in the community. Growth and development surveillance are important. Protect from secondary infections with good handwashing and protective isolation as warranted by CD4 and T-lymphocyte counts. Help keep hydrated, maintain good nutrition, and encourage development as much as tolerated. Administer antibiotics and antifungals as ordered. Provide education about transmission and prevention of HIV infection.

Complications. Failure to thrive or HIV wasting syndrome, loss of developmental milestones, multiple and persistent infections, lymphoid interstitial pneumonitis (LIP), *pneumocystis carinii* pneumonia (PCP), HIV encephalopathy, and death.

Kawasaki Disease

Infective Organism. Unknown. Epidemiologic and clinical features suggest infectious cause.

Sources. No evidence of human-to-human or common-source spread but incidence slightly higher in siblings of clients with this disease.

Incubation Period. Unknown.

Signs and Symptoms. Disease occurs mostly in children <5 year of age. Have fever for ≥5 days and at least four of the following five features, or fever and three of the features and evidence of coronary artery abnormalities. Features appear within several days of onset of fever and include the following: (1) injected bulbar conjunctiva without discharge; (2) red mouth and pharynx, strawberry tongue, and red, cracked lips; (3) generalized rash; (4) peeling and redness of palms and soles; and (5) unilateral cervical lymphadenopathy ≥1.5 cm in diameter.

Isolation. Standard precautions for hospitalized patients.

Nursing Care. Supportive care. Administer anti-inflammatory therapy as ordered. Children usually receive high-dose immune globulin intravenous (IGIV) therapy and high-dose aspirin (80–100 mg/kg/24 hr q.i.d. and then decrease to 3–5 mg/kg/day when fever is under control). Monitor aspirin levels, provide for comfort and nutrition, and be alert to signs and symptoms of congestive heart failure (CHF), murmurs, and arrhythmias.

Complications. Major complication is risk for development of coronary artery aneurysms.

Measles (Rubeola)

Infective Organism. RNA virus classified as morbillivirus.

Sources. Humans.

Transmission. Direct contact with droplets; less commonly airborne.

Incubation Period. Usually 8–12 days.

Period of Communicability. Mainly during prodromal stage and lasting until 4–5 days after rash appears.

Signs and Symptoms. Fever, cough, coryza, conjunctivitis with photophobia, and Koplik's spots on posterior buccal mucosa, followed in 2–3 days by erythematous maculopapular rash beginning on face and spreading downward. Rash is confluent and turns a brownish color after 3–4 days. Skin may peel over heavily rashed areas. Other symptoms include anorexia, general malaise, and general lymphadenopathy.

Isolation. Airborne precautions for 4–5 days after onset of rash. Immunocompromised children need to be isolated for entire course of illness because of prolonged excretion of virus in respiratory secretions.

Nursing Care. Symptomatic. Bedrest, antipyretics, dim lights, cool mist vaporizer, tepid baths.

Complications. Otitis media (OM), bronchopneumonia, croup, and diarrhea in young children; encephalitis; and rarely, subacute sclerosing pa nencephalitis (SSPE).

Mumps

Infective Organism. Paramyxovirus.

Sources. Humans.

Transmission. Direct contact via respiratory route.

Incubation Period. Usually 16–18 days.

Signs and Symptoms. Fever, headache, earache, and malaise followed by swelling and pain of one or both parotid glands, although one-third of infections do not cause apparent salivary swelling.

Isolation. Droplet precautions until 9 days after onset of parotid swelling.

Nursing Care. Supportive. Bedrest, antipyretics, analgesics, increased fluids, soft bland diet, hot or cold compresses to parotid glands.

Complications. Encephalitis (rare) or orchitis (more common in adults).

Pertussis (Whooping Cough)

Infective Organism. *Bordetella pertussis.*

Sources. Humans.

Transmission. Close contact via respiratory secretions.

Incubation Period. 6–20 days, usually 7–10 days.

Signs and Symptoms. Mild upper respiratory symptoms progressing to severe paroxysms of coughing with inspiratory "whoop" usually followed by vomiting. Fever, if present, is usually low grade. In infants <6 months, apnea is a common symptom and whoop is often absent.

Isolation. Droplet precautions for 5 days after beginning effective therapy or until 3 weeks after onset of cough if not treated with antimicrobial therapy.

Nursing Care. Erythromycin is usually drug of choice but others can be used. Supportive care consists of maintaining adequate hydration, administering supplemental oxygen as needed, increasing humidity via humidifier or tent, suctioning nasal secretions, administering inhaled bronchodilators, maintaining quiet bedrest, and vigilant observation for airway obstruction.

Complications. Pneumonia, seizures, hernia, prolapsed rectum, encephalopathy, and death.

Disease is most severe in first year of life, especially for preterm infants.

Rotavirus

Infective Organism. Rotavirus, an RNA virus belonging to the family Reoviridae.

Sources. Humans, mostly and possibly fomites.

Transmission. Fecal-oral route. Found on toys and hard surfaces in day care centers. Also could have respiratory transmission.

Incubation Period. 1–3 days.

Signs and Symptoms. Diarrhea usually preceded or accompanied by vomiting and low-grade fever.

Diagnostic Testing. Enzyme immunoassay (EIA) and latex agglutination assays for group A rotavirus-antigen detection in stool during diarrhea.

Isolation. Strict contact precautions for duration of illness and hospitalization. Prolonged fecal shedding of low concentration of virus after recovery.

Nursing Care. Symptomatic. Prevent dehydration by administering IV fluids as ordered. Good skin care in diaper area. Educate caregiver about good handwashing technique and use of gloves with diaper changes.

Complications. Severe cases can cause dehydration with electrolyte imbalances; acidosis, which can lead to neurologic signs.

Rubella (German Measles, Three-Day Measles)

Infective Organism. RNA virus classified as rubivirus.

Sources. Humans.

Transmission. Direct or droplet contact with nasal secretions. Some infants with congenital rubella shed virus in nasopharyngeal secretions and urine for ≥1 year.

Incubation Period. 14–21 days, but usually 16–18 days.

Period of Communicability. Seven days before to about 5 days after appearance of rash.

Signs and Symptoms. Postnatal: Pinkish-red maculopapular discrete rash beginning on face and progressing rapidly downward; covers body the first day. Disappears in order it came, usually by day 3. Accompanied in older children by low-grade fever and generalized lymphadenopathy, especially suboccipital, cervical, and postauricular. Transient polyarthralgia and polyarthritis common in adolescent girls.

Isolation. Postnatal: Droplet precautions for first 7 days after onset of rash. Congenital: Contact isolation; consider contagious until 1 year old.

Nursing Care. Supportive. Antipyretics for fever and analgesics for discomfort.

Complications. Encephalitis, thrombocytopenia (rare). Biggest complication is teratogenic effect on fetus.

Streptococcal Tonsillitis or Pharyngitis

Infective Organism. Group A β-hemolytic streptococci.

Sources. Humans.

Transmission. Contact with respiratory tract secretions.

Incubation Period. Usually 2–5 days.

Signs and Symptoms. Occurs at all ages but most commonly in school-age children. Present with fever; sore throat; and swollen, tender tonsillar nodes, and can have palatal petechiae and white, strawberry tongue. Tonsils usually swollen and red and have yellow exudate. Toddlers present with moderate fever, serous rhinitis, irritability, and anorexia.

Isolation. Droplet precautions recommended until 24 hours after starting antibiotics.

Nursing Care. Obtain throat swab for rapid strep test or culture as ordered. Make sure to swab both tonsillar pillars and the posterior pharynx, taking care to avoid tongue by using tongue blade. Administer antibiotics as ordered. Severe cases may require treatment with glucocorticoids to decrease inflammation. Provide for comfort measures and fever control p.r.n.

Tuberculosis (TB)

Infective Organism. Mycobacterium tuberculosis.

Sources. Humans; children usually get it from infected adults.

Transmission. Airborne inhalation from infected respiratory droplets from an adult or adolescent with infectious pulmonary tuberculosis.

Incubation Period. From infection to TB skin test being positive is 2–12 weeks. Risk for developing disease state is greatest in first 6 months after infection and remains high for 2 years. Most become dormant.

Signs and Symptoms. Positive Mantoux test using five tuberculin units of purified protein derivative (PPD) administered intradermally indicates infection. Tests should be read 48–72 hours after placement. Positivity interpreted as follows as recommended by the American Academy of Pediatrics Committee on Infectious Diseases (American Academy of Pediatrics, 2000). These recommendations apply regardless of bacille Calmette-Guérin (BCG) vaccine administration.

Reaction ≥5 mm
- Children in close contact with persons with known or suspected infectious TB
- Children suspected to have TB because of positive chest X ray or clinical evidence of TB
- Children with immunosuppressive conditions including immunosuppressive dose of corticosteroids or HIV infection

Reaction ≥10 mm
- Children at increased risk of acquiring TB as a result of the following:
  — Young age (<4 years old)
  — Medical risk factors of Hodgkin's lymphoma, diabetes mellitus, chronic renal failure, malnutrition
- Children with increased environmental exposure:
  — Foreign-born children or children of parents born in regions of increased TB incidence
  — Travel or exposure to high-prevalence regions of the world
- Frequent exposure to adults who are HIV infected; homeless; drug users; or residents of nursing homes, institutions, or prisons or migrant farm workers

Reaction ≥15 mm
- Children ≥4 years old without any risk factors

Most children are asymptomatic. Early manifestations include lymphadenopathy, pulmonary involvement with or without consolidation, pleural effusion, miliary TB, and TB meningitis.

Classifications:

Exposure: Positive recent contact with suspected or confirmed adult with pulmonary TB, negative PPD, normal physical examination (PE), and normal chest X ray.

Infection: Positive PPD in client with normal PE and normal chest X ray or chest X ray with granuloma or calcifications only.

Disease: Positive PPD, signs and symptoms of disease, and positive chest X ray.

Isolation. Most children who are hospitalized require only standard precautions. Those with positive acid-fast bacillus (AFB) in sputum smears should have airborne precautions until after treatment is effective, sputum shows decreasing organisms, and cough is going away.

Nursing Care. Appropriate testing and interpretation. Isolation if necessary. Administer medication as indicated and educate caregivers of importance of compliance with preventive chemotherapy. Preventive chemotherapy usually with isoniazid (INH) 10 mg/kg/day for 6–9 months daily (max. dose: 300 mg). Those with active disease treated with 6-, 9-, or 12-month regimens, depending on site of infection, using combination of two, three, or four of the following drugs: INH, rifampin, pyrazinamide, or streptomycin. Partial treatment can lead to drug resistance. All children with active TB should be tested for HIV. Ensure nutritious meals and adequate rest and monitor growth and development.

Complications. Drug resistance; adverse reactions to drug therapy.

CONGENITAL CARDIAC DEFECTS AND REPAIRS

Presenting signs and symptoms (depending on defect); degree of the following may vary.

History

Poor feeding, decreased weight gain, tiring with feeding, sweating, frequent respiratory infections, fast or hard breathing, inability to keep up with peers, easily fatigued.

Physical Examination

Tachycardia, bradycardia, tachypnea, elevated BP, palpable thrills, decreased pulses, poor perfusion, murmurs; may show symptoms of failure to thrive and lags in development.

Diagnostic Work-up

Chest X ray	To determine heart size and location
Electrocardiogram (ECG)	To measure electrical activity of heart
Holter monitor	24-hour monitoring of heart rate (HR) and rhythm
Echocardiogram (ECHO)	Sound waves show images of heart formations
Cardiac catheterization (Invasive procedure)	Catheter is advanced, usually through femoral vessels, to visualize heart structures and blood flow patterns and to measure pressures and oxygen levels

Common Defects and Repairs

Defects Causing Increase in Pulmonary Blood Flow

Atrial Septal Defect (ASD). Opening between atriums. Usually repaired with surgical Dacron patch closure. Nonsurgical repair using devices during cardiac catheterization is available.

Ventricular Septal Defect (VSD). Opening between ventricles. Can be classified as membranous or muscular. Commonly associated with other defects. Small VSDs are repaired with pursestring suture, large ones with knitted Dacron patch. Nonsurgical repair using devices during cardiac catheterization is available. Many small VSDs close spontaneously in first year of life.

Endocardial Cushion Defect (Arteriovenous [AV] Canal). Low ASD continuous with high VSD and cleft of mitral and tricuspid valves. Palliative treatment is to do a pulmonary artery (PA) banding. Full repair involves patch closure of septal defects and reconstruction of valve tissue. Some need mitral valve replacements.

Patent Ductus Arteriosus (PDA). Condition in which fetal ductus does not close at birth. Can be treated by surgical ligation, with clip closure, or sometimes occluded during heart catheterization. Administration of indomethacin (prostaglandin inhibitor) is done with premature infants to close patent ductus.

Obstructive Defects

Coarctation of Aorta (CoA). Narrowing of aorta at insertion of ductus arteriosus. Surgical repair involves resection with end-to-end anastomosis of aorta or enlargement of constricted section with graft. Nonsurgical treatment includes the use of balloon angioplasty.

Aortic Stenosis (AS). Narrowing or stricture of aortic valve. Can lead to hypertrophy of left ventricle. Treated surgically with aortic valvotomy or valve replacement. Sometimes can dilate narrowed valve with balloon angioplasty in catheterization laboratory (cath. lab).

Pulmonary Stenosis (PS). Narrowing of entrance to pulmonary artery that can lead to right ventricular hypertrophy. *Pulmonary atresia* is a fused valve that allows no blood flow to lungs and can cause hypoplastic right ventricle. Treated with balloon angioplasty in cath. lab or transventricular valvotomy (Brock procedure).

Defects Causing Decrease in Pulmonary Blood Flow

Tetralogy of Fallot (TOF). Consists of four major problems: VSD, PS, overriding aorta, and right ventricular hypertrophy. Palliative treatment with Blalock-Taussig (BT) shunt or modified BT shunt to provide pulmonary blood flow from right or left subclavian arteries. Complete repair preferred and involves closure of VSD, resection of stenosis, and pericardial patch.

Tricuspid Atresia. Failure of tricuspid valve to develop. Palliative treatment is placement of pulmonary-to-systemic shunt to increase blood flow to lungs and a second stage of bidirectional Glenn shunt. Repair done with modified Fontan procedure.

Mixed Defects

Transposition of Great Arteries (TGA) or Transposition of Great Vessels (TGV). Pulmonary artery arises from left ventricle and aorta from right, so there is no communication between systemic and pulmonary circulation. Is incompatible with life without associated mixed defects such as PDA, ASD, or VSD. Palliative treatment with prostaglandin to keep PDA open and with balloon atrial septostomy (Rashkind procedure). Surgical repair involves arterial switch within first weeks of life or Senning procedure with intraatrial baffle using atrial septum. Mustard procedure using prosthetic material can be done with older children. Rastelli procedure used when child has TGA, VSD, and severe PS.

Total Anomalous Pulmonary Venous Connection (TAPVC). Pulmonary veins do not join left atrium. Surgical treatment varies with anatomic defect.

Truncus Arteriosus. Pulmonary artery and aorta did not separate and they override both ventricles. Treated with modified Rastelli procedure.

Hypoplastic Left Heart Syndrome (HLHS). Underdevelopment of left side of heart leading to hypoplastic left ventricle and aortic atresia. Surgical treatment with multiple-stage Norwood procedure or heart transplant during newborn period.

Nursing Care
Preoperative

Assess vital signs and exercise tolerance and provide adequate nutrition and rest. May need to increment care to conserve child's energy. Maintain hydration. Assess for signs and symptoms of CHF: tachycardia, diaphoresis, decreased perfusion, cold extremities, mottling, duskiness, tachypnea >60, retractions, cyanosis, orthopnea, cough, wheezing, failure to thrive, hepatomegaly, edema, or abnormal weight gain. Assess development. Teach caregivers how to care for child at home or to prepare for surgery if imminent. Provide comfort; administer diuretics and cardiac medications as ordered. Neutral temperature environment conserves energy. If postcatheterization, observe for bleeding and assess circulation of involved extremity.

Postoperative

Assess vital signs. Provide for rest and comfort (administer pain medications as ordered), encourage intake of fluids and progressive ambulation, and give emotional support. Observe for the following complications:

Infection—fever; foul-smelling drainage; increased pain

Congestive heart failure (CHF)—dyspnea, cough, tachypnea, retractions, nasal flaring, hepatomegaly, peripheral edema, sacral edema (newborns and infants), tachycardia, sweating, decreased urine output, pale or cool extremities, weight gain, periorbital edema, jugular venous distension (older children)

Cardiac tamponade—Narrowing pulse pressure; tachycardia; dyspnea; cyanosis; apprehension; tripod position

Heart block—usually bradycardia

Post-pericardial syndrome (PPS)—fever; chest pain; irritability

Prepare for discharge by teaching caregiver how to care for child at home and encourage normalcy.

CONJUNCTIVITIS
Brief Description

Inflammation of conjunctiva is termed *conjunctivitis,* also known as *pink eye.* Etiology usually bacterial, viral, allergic, or chemical.

History and Physical Assessment Findings

Examination of external eye reveals diffuse redness of conjunctiva that is more obvious on palpebral surface. Associated watery or purulent discharge, which usually results in crusting of eyelids, especially on wakening. Child reports minimal pain and normal vision. There is normal papillary and red reflexes.

Nursing Care

Goal is to keep eye(s) clean. Ophthalmic medications need to be administered correctly. Topical antibiotic ointment or drops usually prescribed. Accumulated secretions are removed by warm normal saline cleaning. Infection is highly contagious via direct contact. (Strict handwashing and keeping child out of school or day care for 24 hours will help minimize transmission.) Systemic antihistamines prescribed for children with allergic conjunctivitis.

Related Nursing Diagnoses	NOC Outcomes	NIC Interventions
• *Infection*	• Infection status • Knowledge: infection control	• Infection control • Infection protection

CROHN'S DISEASE

Brief Description

Crohn's disease is a chronic inflammatory disease of the bowel. Any portion of the GI tract (from mouth to anus) may be affected. Inflammation involves all layers of the bowel wall and the disease usually occurs segmentally (skip lesions). Terminal ileum is the most frequent site of involvement. Cause is primarily unknown, although infectious, immunologic, environmental, and genetic factors are implicated.

History and Physical Assessment Findings

Abdominal cramping pain, diarrhea, and weight loss are the most common symptoms. Rectal discomfort and perianal disease should be assessed. With disease progression anorexia, malnutrition, anemia, growth retardation, malaise, fever, and fluid or electrolyte disturbances become common. Child and family should be prepared for the following diagnostic tests: sigmoidoscopy, colonoscopy, ultrasonography, barium enema, upper GI series, and CT scanning. Blood tests performed include CBC, sed rate, C-reactive protein, albumin, and electrolyte levels.

Nursing Care

Because the overall goal is to control the inflammatory process, administration of various pharmacological agents is common. These include corticosteroids (such as prednisone), aminosalicylates, sulfasalazine, immunosuppressives (such as methotrexate), and biologic therapies (such as Remicade). Nutritional support (enteral and parenteral nutrition) is a paramount concern since growth failure is a common occurrence. Parents and children should be educated regarding a balanced high-protein, high-calorie diet. Supplemental multivitamins and minerals are often prescribed. In some cases, surgical interventions are necessary (i.e., ileostomy, colectomy).

Related Nursing Diagnoses	NOC Outcomes	NIC Interventions
• *Fluid volume, deficient*	• Fluid balance	• Fluid management • Electrolyte monitoring • Laboratory data interpretation • Total parenteral nutrition • Hemorrhage control
• *Risk for infection*	• Infection status • Safety status: physical injury	• Infection protection • Laboratory data interpretation • Medication administration • Specimen management • Vital signs monitoring
• *Acute pain*	• Comfort level • Pain control	• Pain management • Coping enhancement • Distraction
• *Nausea*	• Comfort level • Hydration • Symptom severity	• Fluid/electrolyte management • Nausea management • Medication management • Vomiting management
• *Diarrhea*	• Electrolyte and acid-base balance • Symptom severity	• Fluid/electrolyte management • Diarrhea management • Laboratory data interpretation • Anxiety reduction • Medication administration
• *Skin integrity, impaired, risk for (perineal/perianal area)*	• Tissue integrity: skin and mucous membranes	• Bathing • Bowel incontinence care • Skin care: topical treatments • Diarrhea management • Perineal care • Self-care assistance • Bathing/hygiene
• *Knowledge, deficient*	• Knowledge: medication • Knowledge: disease process	• Teaching: prescribed medication • Teaching: disease process

CROUP
Brief Description

Croup is a term applied to several viral and bacterial syndromes; however, the most common cause of acute stridor in young children is viral laryngotracheobronchitis (LTB). This upper airway illness results from swelling of structures in the airway and can result in significant airway obstruction. Common pathogens include parainfluenza, RSV, adenovirus, influenza A, and mycoplasma pneumoniae. Croup usually occurs in late fall and winter months and incidence peaks at age 6 months to 3 years.

History and Physical Assessment Findings

Children with croup have a characteristic seal-like, barking cough. Other common symptoms include fever, tachypnea, inspiratory stridor, cough, and hoarseness. Chest X ray may demonstrate steeple sign (i.e., subglottic narrowing). Children with croup may have retractions, mental status changes (especially agitation and restlessness), cyanosis, and low oxygen-saturation levels.

Nursing Care

It is imperative to keep child and family calm. This will help facilitate breathing and oxygenation. Humidification and supplemental oxygen (if saturation <92%) therapy are common interventions. Corticosteroids (e.g., dexamethasone) may be prescribed to decrease airway edema. Nebulized racemic epinephrine and oral dexamethasone are usually prescribed for moderate croup. Children with severe croup are usually prescribed nebulized racemic epinephrine and PO/NG prednisolone. Most children with croup are managed at home unless respiratory distress is severe and warrants frequent monitoring.

Related Nursing Diagnoses	NOC Outcomes	NIC Interventions
• *Breathing pattern, ineffective*	• Respiratory status: airway patency • Respiratory status: ventilation • Vital signs status	• Airway management • Respiratory monitoring • Ventilation assistance • Vital signs monitoring
• *Gas exchange, impaired*	• Respiratory status: gas exchange • Respiratory status: ventilation • Tissue perfusion: pulmonary • Vital signs status	• Acid-base management: respiratory acidosis • Airway management • Oxygen therapy • Respiratory monitoring

(Continued)

Related Nursing Diagnoses	NOC Outcomes	NIC Interventions
• *Fluid volume, deficient, risk for*	• Fluid balance • Hydration • Electrolyte and acid-base balance	• Fluid/electrolyte management • Fluid monitoring • Intravenous therapy
• *Anxiety*	• Anxiety control • Coping	• Anxiety reduction • Coping enhancement
• *Knowledge, deficient*	• Knowledge: disease process, illness care, treatment regimen	• Teaching: procedure and treatment • Teaching: disease process

CYSTIC FIBROSIS (CF)

Brief Description

CF is an inherited autosomal-recessive disorder of the exocrine glands, which causes glands to produce highly viscous secretions of mucus. The mutated gene is located on chromosome 7. Respiratory, gastrointestinal (GI), musculoskeletal, reproductive, and integumentary systems are altered. Ultimately, all organs with mucous ducts become obstructed and damaged. There is a lack of secretion of enzymes from blocked pancreatic ducts leading to altered digestion of fats and proteins. Lungs become filled with mucus, causing air trapping in small airways and eventually leading to recurrent respiratory infections. Males with CF become sterile because of blockage of the vas deferens. Females usually experience infertility resulting from increased mucous secretions in the reproductive tract, interfering with sperm mobility.

History and Physical Assessment Findings

History of meconium ileus or other obstructive bowel diseases may be present in infant. Often these are first indications of CF. Fatty stool, termed *steatorrhea,* is a classic sign of CF. Other common signs and symptoms are chronic or productive cough and frequent respiratory infection. Child often has symptoms of failure to thrive despite strong appetite and commonly falls off growth curve. Definitive diagnosis is made through skin sweat testing (pilocarpine iontophoresis), presence of aforementioned symptoms, or family history. In utero diagnosis is now possible.

Nursing Care

Nursing care is centered on the following activities: maintaining respiratory function, managing or preventing infection, ensuring optimum nutrition, preventing GI blockages, and meeting child's and family's psychosocial needs. Nebulized bronchodilators (e.g., albuterol), aerosol dornase alfa (pulmozyme), anti-inflammatory agents (e.g., steroids, nonsteroidal anti-inflammatory drugs [NSAIDs]), chest physiotherapy, antibiotics, pancreatic enzyme supplements, multivitamin supplements, and dietary supplements are mainstays of treatment. Because of the need for frequent hospitalization, it is important to include caregivers in child's care as much as possible to help maintain child's home routine. Emotional support is essential because this disease affects all members of the family and places constraints on daily activities of all involved.

Related Nursing Diagnoses	NOC Outcomes	NIC Interventions
• *Airway clearance, ineffective*	• Respiratory status: airway patency • Respiratory status: gas exchange • Respiratory status: ventilation • Aspiration control	• Airway management • Airway suctioning • Aspiration precautions • Cough enhancement • Oxygen therapy • Positioning • Respiratory monitoring • Ventilation assistance
• *Risk for infection*	• Infection status • Knowledge: infection control	• Infection control • Infection protection
• *Nutrition, imbalanced: less than body requirements*	• Nutritional status: food and fluid intake • Nutritional status: nutrient intake	• Fluid monitoring • Nutrition management • Nutritional monitoring • Weight gain assistance
• Interrupted family processes	• Family coping • Family functioning • Family health status • Parenting	• Coping enhancement • Family integrity promotion • Family process maintenance • Family support • Normalization promotion

DEPRESSION

Brief Description

Children most at risk for *depression* are those with depressed caregivers, divorced caregivers, recent loss of parent(s), hospitalized siblings, attention deficit disorder (ADD) or ADHD, mild mental retardation, low socioeconomic status, and chronic illness. Classic presentation is child who appears sad; however, depression in children may manifest as hyperactivity and aggression.

History and Physical Assessment Findings

Symptoms often include depressed mood, loss of interest, significant weight loss or gain, insomnia or hypersomnia, fatigue, feelings of worthlessness, tendency to be alone, inappropriate guilt, decreased concentration, and recurrent thoughts of death.

Nursing Care

Seriously depressed children (especially those with suicidal or homicidal ideation) require hospitalization. Outpatient therapy is indicated for those with mild to moderate depression. Referral to mental health professional is necessary. Psychotherapy or pharmacotherapy is often indicated. A variety of pharmacological agents are used to treat childhood depression.

Related Nursing Diagnoses	NOC Outcomes	NIC Interventions
• *Fatigue*	• Activity tolerance • Psychomotor energy	• Mood management • Energy management
• *Sleep pattern disturbed, risk for*	• Comfort level • Rest • Sleep • Well-being	• Sleep enhancement • Coping enhancement
• *Hopelessness*	• Depression control • Depression level • Hope • Quality of life	• Hope instillation • Decision-making support • Mood management • Resiliency promotion
• *Social isolation*	• Social interaction skills • Social involvement • Social support	• Behavior modification: social skills • Complex relationship building • Socialization enhancement

- *Violence: self-directed, risk for*

- Depression control
- Depression level
- Distorted thought control
- Impulse control
- Suicide self-restraint

- Behavior management: self-harm
- Environmental management: violence prevention
- Hope instillation
- Impulse control training
- Suicide prevention

- *Violence: other-directed, risk for*

- Abusive behavior self-control
- Aggression control
- Distorted thought control
- Impulse control
- Risk control: alcohol use
- Risk control: drug use

- Abuse protection support
- Environmental management: violence prevention
- Impulse control training

DERMATITIS
Brief Description

Atopic dermatitis refers to a type of eczema. This inflammatory skin disorder is usually associated with allergy and begins during infancy. Erythema, edema, papules, weeping, scales, and intense pruritus are hallmarks of eczema. *Contact dermatitis* refers to an inflammatory skin reaction to chemical substances resulting in hypersensitivity response. Contact dermatitis is characterized by acute onset of pruritic papulovesicular lesions localized to site of antigen contact. Common causes include poison ivy, oak, sumac and nickel allergy (from jewelry).

History and Physical Assessment
Findings

Atopic dermatitis findings include erythematous papules and vesicles with weeping, oozing, and crusts. Lesions usually found on scalp, forehead, cheeks, forearms, wrists, elbows, and backs of knees. Lesions associated with paroxysmal and intense pruritus. Family history of allergies is common (e.g., asthma, hayfever).

Contact dermatitis develops first as early erythema followed by swelling, urticaria, or maculopapular vesicles and scales. Often accompanied by intense pruritus.

Nursing Care

Atopic dermatitis: Goals of management include relieving pruritus, hydrating skin, reducing inflammation, and preventing secondary infection. Cool, wet compresses are soothing to skin. Aveeno oatmeal baths are useful in relieving pruritus. Antihistamines such as hydroxyzine hydrochloride (Atarax) and diphenhydramine hydrochloride (Benadryl) may also be prescribed. Skin emollients such as Eucerin cream are often used to hydrate skin. Families should be instructed to avoid hot baths and scented soaps. Topical steroids such as hydrocortisone ointment, triamcinolone, or fluocinonide (Lidex) may be ordered. New nonsteroidal topical treatment with immunomodulators (i.e., Tacrolimus, Pimecrolimus) may also be prescribed. Fingernails should be kept short and clean to prevent infection. Lesions should be examined for signs of infection (honey-colored crusting with surrounding erythema) and reported to health care practitioner.

Contact dermatitis: Teach client regarding need to avoid further contact with allergen. Topical steroid preparations usually ordered. Oral antihistamines may be prescribed to alleviate itching. Oral steroids (e.g., prednisone) usually ordered if lesions are on face or genitals, if they are widespread, or if there is generalized edema. Fingernails should be kept short and clean to prevent infection. Lesions should be examined for signs of infection (e.g., increased erythema, linear streaking) and reported to health care practitioner.

Related Nursing Diagnoses	NOC Outcomes	NIC Interventions
• *Skin integrity, impaired*	• Tissue integrity: skin and mucous membranes	• Skin surveillance • Wound care
• *Risk for infection*	• Infection status • Knowledge: infection control	• Infection control • Infection protection

DIABETES MELLITUS (TYPE 1 AND TYPE 2)

Brief Description

Type 1 (previously known as insulin-dependent) *diabetes mellitus* (DM) is the most common chronic metabolic disorder in the pediatric population. Type 1 DM results in hyperglycemia usually secondary to insulin deficiency from the loss of pancreas beta cell functioning and insulin production. This results in high blood sugar and other problems with carbohydrate and fat metabolism. The mode of inheritance is still not well described. However, evidence suggests that genetic predisposition is an important factor. Viral infection is thought to be a significant antecedent. This type of antecedent is thought to initiate an autoimmune process that gradually destroys beta cells. Diabetic ketoacidosis (DKA) is a metabolic state characterized by acidosis, elevated serum glucose, and serum ketones. DKA may be precipitated by physical or emotional stress, infection, and noncompliance with insulin therapy. Often, DKA is the first presentation of Type 1 DM in children.

There has been a significant increase in the number of children diagnosed with Type 2 (previously known as noninsulin-dependent) diabetes mellitus. Obesity and sedentary lifestyle are strong risk factors for Type 2 DM. Type 2 DM is characterized by insulin resistance; there is a relative, not absolute, deficiency of insulin. Because of insulin resistance, the body fails to use insulin appropriately. African Americans, Mexican Americans, Asian Americans, and Native Americans are at highest risk.

History and Physical Assessment Findings

Type 1—History generally reveals cardinal signs and symptoms of weight loss, polydipsia, polyphagia, and polyuria. Other physical examination findings are usually within normal limits unless child is in DKA. Children in DKA appear weak and lethargic, progressing to comatose (considered a medical emergency). Signs and symptoms of severe dehydration are often present. Breath may have fruity odor and Kussmaul respirations may be present. Laboratory tests demonstrate elevated fasting blood sugar and postprandiol glucose levels. Oral glucose tolerance test (OGTT) may be ordered to confirm the diagnosis.

Type 2—Often, children with Type 2 DM are asymptomatic. Usually, these children have hypertension, dyslipidemia, and are obese. Type 2 DM is diagnosed by fasting blood glucose levels, postprandial plasma glucose levels, and oral glucose tolerance test.

Nursing Care

Multidisciplinary focus of care is necessary (i.e., pediatric endocrinologist, diabetes nurse educator, nutritionist, social worker, school nurse). For children with Type 1 DM, insulin therapy remains the hallmark of treatment. Children are generally prescribed two daily doses of subcutaneous insulin (combination of regular and intermediate or long-acting types). More intensive insulin dosages (>2 injections per day or continuous SC infusion via insulin pump) may be prescribed. Recent research has demonstrated that tight control with intensive insulin therapy is associated with fewer long-term complications of DM. Children and caregivers are taught about insulin administration (i.e., mixing insulins, drawing up dosages, injection sites). Urine ketones are monitored if glucose levels are >250 mg/dL or if the child is sick. Children with

Type 2 DM are managed by weight control or reduction, exercise, and dietary modifications. Oral hypoglycemic agents may also be prescribed.

Children and families are also taught how to perform self-blood glucose monitoring. Diet counseling is required; consistency of mealtimes is a paramount concern. Exercise is promoted. Signs, symptoms, and treatment of hypoglycemia and hyperglycemia are taught to caregivers and children. Psychological support to assist in coping with this lifelong chronic illness is necessary.

Diabetic ketoacidosis (DKA) is a life-threatening condition and is treated as a medical emergency, usually in the pediatric intensive care unit (PICU). Because of the severe electrolyte and fluid imbalances, metabolic acidosis, and cerebral edema, this condition is managed precisely and carefully. Collaborative care is required in order to restore the normal pH level, correct fluid and electrolyte balance, restore normal blood glucose, decrease cerebral edema, and lower increased intracranial pressure (ICP).

Medical treatment includes fluid resuscitation and electrolyte replacement. In cases of hypovolemic shock, boluses of intravenous (IV) fluids may be given at a rate of 10–20 mL/kg. Potassium chloride is administered in doses dependent upon serum K levels (once renal function or urine output is confirmed). For example, in select situations, doses up to 40 mEq/L may be administered in 1 hour. Continuous EKG monitoring is warranted to assess for life-threatening cardiac arrhythmias. Bicarbonate is no longer used in treating DKA because of the increased risk of metabolic acidosis and hyperosmolality.

A continuous infusion of regular insulin is administered via infusion pump, usually at a rate of .05–.1 units/kg/hr. However, serum glucose levels should not be lowered rapidly due to the risk of cerebral edema. Insulin is carefully titrated to decrease the serum glucose level at a rate not to exceed 100 mg/dL/hr. Intravenous regular insulin is tapered off and the child is transitioned to doses of subcutaneous insulin when stable.

Related Nursing Diagnoses	NOC Outcomes	NIC Interventions
• *Knowledge, deficient*	• Knowledge: diabetes management	• Teaching: prescribed diet, disease process, prescribed activity/ exercise, prescribed medication, psychomotor skill
• *Nutrition, impaired: less than body requirements*	• Nutritional status • Weight control	• Nutrition management • Nutrition monitoring

(Continued)

- *Fluid volume, deficient*
  - Electrolyte and acid-base balance
  - Fluid balance
  - Hydration
  - Nutritional status: food and fluid intake
  - Electrolyte/fluid management
  - Fluid monitoring
  - Hypovolemic management
  - Intravenous therapy
  - Shock management, volume

- *Risk for infection*
  - Immune status
  - Infection status
  - Knowledge: infection control
  - Risk detection
  - Health screening
  - Immunization/vaccination management
  - Infection control
  - Infection protection
  - Wound care

- *Home maintenance, impaired*
  - Family functioning
  - Self-care
  - Family integrity promotion

- *Noncompliance, risk for*
  - Adherence behavior
  - Compliance behavior
  - Symptom control
  - Mutual goal setting
  - Self-modification assistance
  - Self-responsibility facilitation
  - Teaching: disease process

- *Family processes, readiness for enhanced*
  - Family functioning
  - Family health status
  - Family integration promotion
  - Family support

EATING DISORDERS
ANOREXIA NERVOSA

Brief Description

Anorexia nervosa (AN) is characterized by refusal to maintain minimally normal body weight. Usually includes significant fear of being overweight. Child experiences hunger but denies it. More prevalent in middle- and upper-class white females. Mean age of onset is 13–14 years. Often described as perfectionists and high achievers. Have disturbed perception of body size even when significantly underweight. Most often, AN presents as a lifelong problem.

History and Physical Assessment Findings

Symptoms include weight loss of >15% body weight, amenorrhea, sleep disturbances, denial of illness, arrested pubertal progression, obvious cachexia, hypothermia, bradycardia, hypotension, scalp hair loss, electrolyte imbalances, and ECG abnormalities.

Nursing Care

Outpatient treatment usually recommended for those who have had the disease <4 months. Family functioning should be intact for those receiving outpatient treatment. Those with severe weight loss, starvation, drug use, abnormal ECG, or severe depression should receive inpatient treatment. Interdisciplinary care with mental health professionals, health care practitioners, social workers, nurses, and nutritionists is necessary. Nutritional therapy, psychotherapy, or behavior therapy regimens are used.

EATING DISORDERS
BULIMIA

Brief Description

Bulimia nervosa (BN) is a disorder characterized by binge eating in association with self-induced vomiting, severe food restriction, cathartic or laxative abuse, strenuous exercise, or heightened concern with body shape. Binge eaters usually are unaware of being hungry before eating but cannot stop once they start. Classified as a type of addiction. Episodes of binging and purging are accompanied by depressed mood and awareness of abnormal eating pattern. Those with career aspirations that require low weight (e.g., athletics, modeling) are most at risk.

History and Physical Assessment Findings

History usually reveals that disorder began with only occasional episodes of binging and purging. With progression of disease, frequency of binging and purging and amount of food intake increases; loss of control over behaviors is gradual. Frequency of binging and purging varies from 1x/week to many times per day. Fluid and electrolyte loss is common. May also have diminished reflexes secondary to potassium depletion and cardiac arrhythmias. Laboratory tests often reveal anemia. Erosion of tooth enamel, dental caries, esophagitis, sore throat, and parotitis are often findings related to repeated self-induced vomiting and irritation from stomach acid. Backs of hands may be scarred or cut from teeth during self-induced vomiting.

Nursing Care

Management of BN involves medical, psychologic, behavioral, and nutritional components. Hospitalization is required for those with fluid and electrolyte imbalances and cardiac complications. Outpatient therapy involves nutritional consultation and behavioral therapy. Psychopharmacologic interventions have been effective in reducing the urge to binge and vomit. Home environment should be structured so as to reduce potential for binging behavior; includes eliminating binge-type foods (e.g., high-caloric sweets) and restricting eating to one room in the home. Telephone support has been demonstrated to be useful.

Related Nursing Diagnoses	NOC Outcomes	NIC Interventions
• *Health maintenance, ineffective*	• Health-seeking behavior • Participation: health care decisions • Psychosocial adjustment: life change • Self-direction of care • Social support • Treatment behavior: illness	• Health system guidance • Decision-making support • Family involvement promotion • Self-modification assistance • Self-responsibility facilitation • Support group • Support system enhancement
• *Nutrition, imbalanced: less than body requirements*	• Nutrition status: food, fluid, and nutrient intake • Weight control	• Eating disorders management • Nutrition management • Nutritional monitoring • Weight gain assistance
• *Fluid volume, deficient, risk for*	• Electrolyte and acid-base balance • Nutritional status: food and fluid intake	• Fluid/electrolyte management • Fluid monitoring • IV therapy • Nutrition management
• *Ineffective coping*	• Coping • Decision making • Role performance	• Coping enhancement • Decision-making support • Role enhancement • Support group • Support system enhancement
• *Self-mutilation*	• Self-mutilation restraint	• Behavior management: self-harm
• *Thought processes, disturbed*	• Distorted thought control	• Delusion management • Environmental management: safety
• *Hypothermia, risk for*	• Thermoregulation	• Temperature regulation • Hypothermia treatment *(Continued)*

Related Nursing Diagnoses	NOC Outcomes	NIC Interventions
• *Disturbed body image*	• Body image • Distorted thought control • Self-esteem	• Body image enhancement • Self-esteem enhancement
• *Interrupted family processes*	• Family coping • Family functioning • Family health status • Parenting	• Family integrity promotion • Coping enhancement • Family process maintenance • Family support • Parenting promotion
• *Growth and development, delayed, risk for*	• Child development: adolescence • Growth • Physical maturation: female • Physical maturation: male	• Developmental enhancement: adolescent • Nutrition therapy • Nutritional monitoring • Weight management
• *Self-esteem, chronic low*	• Depression level • Self-esteem • Quality of life	• Self-esteem enhancement
• *Dentition, impaired**	• Oral health	• Oral health maintenance • Oral health restoration

*Applicable to bulimia nervosa

EPIGLOTTITIS
Brief Description

Epiglottitis is an inflammation of the epiglottis and constitutes a pediatric emergency. Edema in this area of the airway can progress rapidly, leading to airway obstruction by occlusion of the trachea and epiglottis. Causative organism is often *Haemophilus influenza* type B (Hib). Incidence has decreased since the advent of Hib vaccine. Affects children from 6 months to 10 years of age (average age is 3 year old).

History and Physical Assessment Findings

History is usually consistent with previously healthy child who *suddenly* becomes ill. Onset is abrupt, child often deteriorates quickly, demonstrating

severe signs of respiratory distress. Usually report of fever, sore throat, muffled or hoarse voice, and swallowing difficulty. Stridor worsens as larynx
swells. Child often observed drooling and assumes tripod (i.e., leaning forward with jaw thrusted forward) posture refusing to lay down. X ray reveals
enlarged epiglottis and narrowed airway. Positive blood culture found in
most clients with epiglottitis.

Nursing Care

Airway management, medication administration, hydration, and support are
vital aspects of care. *Visual inspection of the mouth and throat are contraindicated because irritation and hypersensitivity of the airway can lead to
laryngospasm and necessary tracheostomy.* Emergency equipment for intu-
bation and airway maintenance should be readily available. Child should be
kept well oxygenated and calm. Children with epiglottitis are initially managed in pediatric intensive care unit. IV antibiotics (e.g., cefotaxime, ceftriaxone) are given to treat infection, and IV fluids are administered to provide
hydration.

Related Nursing Diagnoses	NOC Outcomes	NIC Interventions
• *Airway clearance, ineffective*	• Respiratory status: airway patency • Respiratory status: gas exchange • Respiratory status: ventilation	• Airway management • Oxygen therapy • Positioning • Respiratory monitoring • Ventilation assistance
• *Risk for infection*	• Infection status	• Infection control • Infection protection
• *Gas exchange, impaired*	• Respiratory status: gas exchange • Respiratory status: ventilation • Tissue perfusion: pulmonary • Vital signs status	• Airway management • Laboratory data interpretation • Oxygen therapy • Respiratory monitoring • Ventilation assistance • Vital signs monitoring
• *Hyperthermia*	• Thermoregulation	• Vital signs monitoring • Fever treatment • Temperature regulation
• *Fear*	• Fear control • Anxiety control	• Anxiety reduction • Coping enhancement

GASTROESOPHAGEAL REFLUX (GER)

Brief Description

GER involves the passive return of stomach contents into the esophagus. This results from increased relaxation of the lower esophageal sphincter. Factors that cause this relaxation include gastric distension, coughing, and obstructive lung disease. GERD (gastroesophageal reflux disease) represents symptoms or tissue damage as a result of GER. This disorder results in passive vomiting and may lead to complications such as pneumonia (especially in young infants), apnea (especially in young infants), esophagitis, and midepigastric pain. The majority of cases resolve by age 6–12 months with the introduction of solid foods.

History and Physical Assessment Findings

History usually reveals a report of passive emesis after feedings. Child may demonstrate poor weight gain (fall off growth curve) in more severe cases. Child may have anemia as a result of bleeding from esophageal mucosa. History of multiple respiratory infections should alert provider to the possibility of GERD. A barium swallow may demonstrate reflux following swallowing. Esophageal pH monitoring is positive if pH is acidic.

Nursing Care

Small, frequent feedings with thickened formula (rice cereal, 1 tsp/1 oz formula) may be recommended. Maintenance of prone, elevated position after feeding is also recommended. Scientific research regarding the effectiveness of these interventions is still inconclusive, although this remains the standard in practice.

Pharmacologic agents such as H_2 antagonists (e.g., Tagamet, Zantac, Pepcid) and proton-pump inhibitors (e.g., Nexium, Prevacid, Prilosec, Protonix) may be prescribed, especially in children with poor weight gain or frequent respiratory infections. Medications such as Reglan may be used to increase the LES pressure and increase gastric emptying time. Surgical treatment (i.e., Nissen fundoplication) is reserved for very severe cases.

Related Nursing Diagnoses	NOC Outcomes	NIC Interventions
• *Nutrition, imbalanced: less than body requirements*	• Nutritional status: food and fluid intake • Nutritional status: nutrient intake • Weight control	• Nutrition management • Weight gain assistance • Positioning

(Continued)

- *Knowledge, deficient*
- Knowledge
- Teaching: disease process
- Teaching: infant nutrition
- Teaching: prescribed diet
- Teaching: procedure and treatment

HIRSCHSPRUNG'S DISEASE

Brief Description

Also known as congenital aganglionic megacolon, *Hirschsprung's disease* is a mechanical intestinal obstruction caused by inadequate motility. Ganglionic cells are absent in one or more segments of the colon. Usually involves the rectum and large intestine. Lack of enervation causes functional defect, and there is lack of peristalsis, which causes accumulation of bowel contents and distension. Ischemia may occur with resulting enterocolitis, which can lead to death.

History and Physical Assessment Findings

In neonates, history of not passing meconium is often found. Neonate may also refuse fluids. Infants generally portray history of failure to thrive, constipation, and abdominal distension. Symptoms during childhood are more chronic in nature and include constipation, ribbon-like stools, and visible peristalsis. Medical diagnosis confirmed by X ray, barium enema, and rectal biopsy.

Nursing Care

Medical treatment usually involves surgery to remove aganglionic portion of colon. Temporary colostomy is often performed to relieve obstruction. Ostomy is usually closed during second surgery when aganglionic portion is removed.

Because enterocolitis is a potential complication, vital signs should be monitored frequently to assess for signs of shock. Fluids and electrolytes are often replaced. Bowel assessments should be performed to detect symptoms of perforation (e.g., fever, increasing distension, irritablility, vomiting). Abdominal girth measurements are often performed to detect progressing distension.

Related Nursing Diagnoses	NOC Outcomes	NIC Interventions
• *Acute pain*	• Comfort level • Pain control • Pain: disruptive effects • Pain level	• Pain management • Medication management • Teaching: procedure and treatment • Distraction • Positioning

(Continued)

Related Nursing Diagnoses	NOC Outcomes	NIC Interventions
• *Risk for infection*	• Infection status • Wound healing	• Infection control • Infection protection • Incision site care • Wound care
• *Anxiety*	• Anxiety control	• Anxiety reduction • Presence • Calming technique
• *Skin integrity, impaired, risk for*	• Tissue integrity: skin • Wound healing	• Skin surveillance • Wound care • Incision site care
• *Knowledge, deficient*	• Knowledge	• Teaching: disease process, preoperative, prescribed medication, procedure and treatment, psychomotor skill
• *Fluid volume, deficient, risk for*	• Fluid balance • Hydration	• Fluid management • Fluid monitoring • Fluid/electrolyte management • Intravenous therapy

IMPETIGO

Brief Description

Impetigo is a highly contagious bacterial infection of the skin. *S. aureus* is the most common causative organism. This vesicular-type lesion spreads peripherally in sharply marginated irregular outlines. Tends to heal without scarring unless secondary infections occur. Easily spread by self-inoculation, and therefore children should be advised to avoid touching involved area. Most common in infants and young children.

History and Physical Assessment Findings

Be alert to history of lesions that begin as red macules and then become vesicular. Lesions are moist vesicles that rupture to form thick, honey-colored crusting. Most commonly located around mouth and nose. Pruritus is common. Child usually asymptomatic; systemic effects are minimal.

Nursing Care

Topical antibiotic cream (e.g., mupirocin [Bactroban]) may be prescribed. Topical treatment usually prescribed for 1 week to 10 days. Children who have widespread lesions and are systemically ill may be prescribed oral antibiotics (e.g., cephalexin or cloxacillin). Area should be gently cleansed with warm water. Caregivers should be taught about the highly contagious nature of this infection. Handwashing is a paramount concern. Other family members should be assessed.

Related Nursing Diagnoses	NOC Outcomes	NIC Interventions
• *Skin integrity, impaired*	• Tissue integrity: skin	• Skin surveillance • Wound care
• *Acute pain*	• Comfort level • Pain control • Pain level	• Analgesic administration • Pain management • Medication management
• *Knowledge, deficient*	• Knowledge	• Teaching: disease process, prescribed medication, procedure and treatment
• *Risk for infection*	• Infection status • Knowledge: infection control	• Infection control • Infection protection • Wound care

IRON DEFICIENCY ANEMIA
Brief Description
Inadequate supply of dietary iron is the most common cause of *iron deficiency anemia*. This is the most prevalent nutritional disorder in the United States. Both young children and adolescents are at risk. Major decrease in incidence has been linked to programs such as Women, Infants, and Children (WIC), although it is still a major health problem in children, especially those from low-income families. Other causes of iron deficiency anemia include impaired absorption of iron, blood loss, excessive demands for iron, and inability to form hemoglobin.

History and Physical Assessment Findings
Signs and symptoms of iron deficiency anemia are most often not obvious. Some common signs are low weight, paleness, tachycardia, positive guaiac test, poor muscle development, and "spoon" nail. History often reveals increased ingestion of milk and poor dietary intake of iron rich foods. Blood analyses reveal hypochromic, microcytic red blood cells (RBCs); low mean corpuscular volume (MCV) and mean corpuscular hemoglobin concentration (MCHC); low reticulocyte count; and low serum ferritin.

Nursing Care

Aim of treatment is to correct cause of anemia. Most often involves dietary counseling. Oral iron supplements usually prescribed. Important to assess compliance with medication administration. Caregivers should be taught proper administration techniques, which include avoiding administration with milk or other products high in phosphorus. Administration of iron with citrus fruit or juice aids in absorption of iron.

Related Nursing Diagnoses	NOC Outcomes	NIC Interventions
• *Nutrition, imbalanced: less than body requirements*	• Nutritional status: nutrient intake	• Nutrition management
• *Health maintenance, ineffective*	• Health-seeking behavior • Knowledge: health behavior • Knowledge: treatment regimen	• Health education • Health screening • Health system guidance • Teaching: procedure and treatment

LEAD POISONING
Brief Description

Lead in paint is the most common source of *lead poisoning* in young children. Ingestion of contaminated food, water, and soil can also lead to lead exposure. African American children living in inner cities represent the largest number of children with lead poisoning. Children absorb and retain more lead proportionately to their weight than adults, putting them at greater risk of poisoning.

History and Physical Assessment Findings

History usually reveals environmental exposure to lead. Clinical manifestations will vary depending on lead level. Children with lead poisoning may be asymptomatic. However, those with moderate to high lead levels may demonstrate learning or behavior problems, irritability, anorexia, malaise, headache, abdominal pain, and vomiting. Those with severe lead poisoning may experience clumsiness, encephalopathy, coma, convulsions, and signs of increased IP.

Nursing Care

Interventions aimed at removing sources of lead in the child's environment are necessary. Treatment consists of chelation therapy as agents bind with lead leading to increased excretion. Agents such as calcium disodium ethylenediaminetetraacetic acid ($CaNa_2$ EDTA), dimercaprol (BAL), and D-penicillamine or dimercaptosuccinic acid (DMSA) are often used. Nursing care should also be aimed at screening, prevention, and education. Caregivers need to understand the importance of follow-up testing. Home health care referrals or social work referral may be appropriate. Current Center for Disease Control (CDC) recommendations include:

Blood Level	Recommendation
<10	Reassess in 1 year or sooner if exposure status changes
10–14	Provide patient and family with lead poisoning education, follow-up testing, and necessary social service referrals
15–19	Provide patient and family with lead poisoning education, follow-up testing, and necessary social service referrals; if level persists initiate actions listed for level of 20–44
20–44	Provide care coordination, clinical management, environmental investigation, and lead hazard control
45–69	Within 48 hours, provide coordination of care and clinical management including chelation therapy, environmental investigation, and lead hazard control (child is not to remain in lead hazard environment)
>70	Immediate provision of medical treatment and chelation therapy, begin coordination of care, environmental investigation, and lead hazard control

Related Nursing Diagnoses	NOC Outcomes	NIC Interventions
• *Poisoning, risk for*	• Medication response • Risk control • Safety behavior: home physical environment	• Environmental management, safety • Surveillance, safety
• *Knowledge, deficient*	• Knowledge	• Teaching: disease process
• *Constipation, risk for*	• Bowel elimination • Hydration	• Constipation or impaction management
• *Nutrition, imbalance: less than body requirements*	• Nutritional status	• Nutrition management • Nutrition monitoring
• *Sensory perception, disturbed, risk for*	• Cognitive orientation • Cognitive ability	• Cognitive stimulation • Nutrition management • Surveillance, safety

OBSESSIVE-COMPULSIVE DISORDER (OCD)

Brief Description

OCD is characterized by repetitive actions that the child knows are abnormal. Often, repetitive handwashing or certain words said before performing a task are symptoms exhibited by the child. Children with OCD may have obsessive thoughts about fear of harm, illness, death, and wrongdoing.

History and Physical Assessment Findings

Classic sign of OCD is child's understanding that the repetitive actions are abnormal and thoughts irrational.

Nursing Care

Management of child with OCD involves behavior modification, psychopharmacologic intervention, and psychotherapy.

Related Nursing Diagnoses	NOC Outcomes	NIC Interventions
• Fatigue	• Activity tolerance • Energy conservation	• Energy management
• Thought processes, disturbed	• Distorted thought control	• Cognitive restructuring

ORBITAL CELLULITIS

Brief Description

Orbital cellulitis is the infection of orbital contents posterior to orbital septum. Usually spreads from adjacent infection of sinus. Common organisms are S. aureus, group A streptococci, S. pneumoniae, and H. influenzae type B.

History and Physical Assessment Findings

Symptoms often include obvious lid edema, pain on eye movement, decreased ocular mobility, and decreased visual acuity. History often reveals sinus congestion or infection.

Nursing Care

Patient hospitalized for IV antibiotics. Ophthalmology referral should be made. Cultures should be obtained. Child needs to be prepared for diagnostic studies such as computed tomography (CT) scan of orbit and sinus. Surgical intervention may be necessary. Need to assess for signs and symptoms of meningeal irritation because risk of bacterial meningitis is increased in those with orbital cellulitis.

Related Nursing Diagnoses	NOC Outcomes	NIC Interventions
• *Risk for infection*	• Infection status • Knowledge: infection control	• Infection control • Infection protection • Wound care
• *Acute pain*	• Comfort level • Pain control	• Analgesic administration • Medication management • Pain management
• *Sensory perception, disturbed*	• Sensory function: vision • Vision compensation behavior	• Communication enhancement: visual deficit • Environmental management

OSTEOMYELITIS

Brief Description

Osteomyelitis represents an infection of the bone. Any bone can be affected but femoral and tibial metaphyses are most commonly involved. Results come from either hematogenous spread (preexisting infection elsewhere) or exogenous (invasion of bone from outside body). Common pathogens are *S. aureus*, group A streptococci, *H. influenzae, Pseudomonas* organisms, and *Salmonella* organisms.

History and Physical Assessment Findings

Child may have history of trauma or fever. Often report limp or inability to bear weight. Affected limb looks swollen, bruised, red, hot, and tender. Child often febrile and irritable and appears systemically ill. Laboratory tests reveal elevated WBCs and erythrocyte sedimentation rate (ESR). Positive blood culture and positive culture of aspirate from involved bone.

Nursing Care

One of the first priorities of care is prompt administration of IV antibiotics. Antibiotic therapy is usually indicated for several weeks. Caregivers may be taught home administration using a central venous catheter. Child is maintained on bed rest with affected extremity immobilized (may need splint or cast). Bed rest and immobilization help prevent the spread of infection.

Surgical interventions may be required in certain cases. Positioning and comfort measures are necessary. Physical therapy consult often initiated as child begins to increase mobility.

Related Nursing Diagnoses	NOC Outcomes	NIC Interventions
• *Risk for infection*	• Infection status • Knowledge: infection control • Wound healing	• Infection control • Infection protection • Incision site care • Wound care
• *Acute pain*	• Comfort level • Pain control • Pain: disruptive effects • Pain level	• Analgesic administration • Medication management • Pain management • Patient-controlled analgesia (PCA) assistance
• *Hyperthermia*	• Thermoregulation	• Fever treatment • Temperature regulation • Vital signs monitoring
• *Tissue perfusion, ineffective, bone*	• Tissue perfusion: bone	• Bone perfusion promotion
• *Mobility: physical, impaired*	• Mobility level	• Positioning • Exercise therapy
• *Knowledge, deficient*	• Knowledge	• Teaching: disease process, prescribed activity/exercise, prescribed medication, psychomotor skill

OTITIS MEDIA (OM)

Brief Description

OM, an inflammation of the middle ear, represents one of the most prevalent diseases in young children. Results from dysfunctioning eustachian tube and often is first childhood illness confronted by caregivers. Incidence greatest in children age 6 months to 2 years and is higher in winter months. Children exposed to environmental tobacco smoke also have higher incidence. *S. pneumoniae* and *H. influenzae* are most common pathogens. Viral agents identified in approximately 40% of cases.

History and Physical Assessment Findings

Otoscopic examination reveals red tympanic membrane (often bulging) with no visible landmarks. History reveals ear pain as evidenced by pulling on ear, fever, irritability, poor PO intake, or associated upper respiratory infection. Culture and sensitivity are not routinely performed, but if drainage is present it will help guide treatment. Other diagnostic tests that may be performed: pneumatic otoscopy, tympanometry, or tympanocentesis.

Nursing Care

A variety of antibiotics are used to treat OM. Amoxicillin remains the first-line drug. Compliance by caregiver and child with antibiotic administration should be assessed. Other commonly prescribed antibiotics are amoxicillin/clavulanate (Augmentin), cefixime (Suprax), erythromycin (Pediazole), cefuroxime (Ceftin), and cotrimoxazole (Bactrim). Conservative antibiotic use is recommended to prevent drug-resistant organisms. Analgesics or antipyretics such as Tylenol and Motrin are also used to treat fever or discomfort. Decongestants and antihistamines have not proven effective.

Related Nursing Diagnoses	NOC Outcomes	NIC Interventions
• Acute pain	• Comfort level • Pain control	• Analgesic administration • Medication management • Pain management
• Risk for infection	• Infection status	• Infection control • Infection protection
• Sensory perception, disturbed	• Hearing compensation behavior	• Communication enhancement: hearing deficit

PEDICULOSIS CAPITIS (HEAD LICE)
Brief Description

Pediculosis capitis is a parasitic infection of the scalp by the louse. Lice infestations are highly communicable. Eggs or nits are at the junction of the hair shaft close to the skin. Head lice are spread by hair-to-hair contact, clothing, and brushes. Louse cannot fly and is transmitted from person to person via personal items. Child may have psychologic effects because infection can be highly stressful to child and family.

History and Physical Assessment Findings

Scalp pruritus with erythema and excoriations is common. Live lice and nits may be seen on hair shaft. Lice are visible to the naked eye as small, grayish dots. Nits appear as whitish specks visible approximately 1/4 inch from scalp and may look like dandruff.

Nursing Care

The pediculicide of choice is Nix crème rinse, which can be purchased over the counter. Ovide (Malathion) is another product available by prescription. Manual removal of nits with a fine-tooth comb is also necessary. Care of the environment is necessary (e.g., washing clothing and bed linens in hot water, vacuuming carpets, boiling hair-care items for 10 min). Children should be taught not to share hair-care items such as combs and barrettes nor caps and other items worn near hair.

Related Nursing Diagnoses	NOC Outcomes	NIC Interventions
• *Risk for infection*	• Infection status • Knowledge: infection control	• Infection protection • Infection control
• *Knowledge, deficient*	• Knowledge	• Teaching: prescribed medication • Teaching: procedure and treatment
• *Self-esteem, risk for situational low*	• Self-esteem	• Self-esteem enhancement

PNEUMONIA

Brief Description

Pneumonia is an infection and inflammation of the lower respiratory tract, specifically of the bronchioles and alveolar spaces of the lungs. Etiology may be viral, bacterial, or mycoplasmal. End-result of pathogen invasion results in accumulation of exudates, which fill alveolar spaces, and consolidation of lung areas.

History and Physical Assessment Findings

History may include acute or subacute onset of symptoms. Symptoms of fever (with chills), cough, dyspnea, tachypnea, shallow breathing, and crackles are common. X ray findings of consolidation confirm diagnosis, although most children are diagnosed by clinical symptoms. CBC results reveal elevated WBCs.

Nursing Care

Most children are managed at home but inpatient therapy is required for those with significant infection and respiratory distress. Ongoing respiratory assessments are indicated. Prescription of anti-infectives depends on the type of pneumonia. Pain management may be necessary, especially during coughing and deep breathing. Antipyretics may be necessary to control fever. Providing adequate hydration is also priority of care.

Related Nursing Diagnoses	NOC Outcomes	NIC Interventions
• *Gas exchange, impaired*	• Respiratory status: gas exchange • Vital signs status	• Oxygen therapy • Acid-base monitoring • Positioning • Energy management • Respiratory monitoring • Vital signs monitoring
• *Airway clearance, ineffective*	• Respiratory status: ventilation • Respiratory status: gas exchange	• Respiratory monitoring • Chest physiotherapy • Positioning • Airway suctioning • Cough enhancement • Medication administration: inhalation
• *Fluid volume, deficient, risk for*	• Fluid balance: hydration	• Fluid management • Fluid monitoring • Intravenous therapy
• *Risk for infection*	• Infection status	• Infection control • Infection prevention • Aspiration precautions • Environmental management: infection control • Cough enhancement
• *Health maintenance, ineffective*	• Knowledge: treatment regimen	• Teaching: disease process • Teaching: procedure and treatment

POST-TRAUMATIC STRESS DISORDER (PTSD)
Brief Description
Children with *PTSD* have a history of exposure to an adverse event thought to be distressing to nearly everyone. Trauma may be persistently reexperienced. Often, these types of events include life-threatening events to self or significant others; death of a loved one; serious injury; physical coercion; an accident; assault; disasters (e.g., flood, plane crash, terrorism, hurricane);

sexual abuse; or witnessing homicide, suicide, or shooting. Risk for PTSD is higher in children who experience more than one of these events.

History and Physical Assessment Findings

Children with PTSD often report difficulty with sleeping, nightmares, anxiety, difficulty with interpersonal relationships, phobias, and agitation.

Nursing Care

Children who experience any traumatic event need to learn how to deal with their emotions. Type of management depends on intensity of event and individual reactions to it. Often, psychologic intervention by a mental health professional is necessary.

Related Nursing Diagnoses	NOC Outcomes	NIC Interventions
• *Post-trauma syndrome*	• Coping • Abuse cessation and protection • Abuse recovery • Fear control • Self-mutilation restraint	• Counseling • Support system enhancement • Security enhancement • Rape-trauma treatment • Coping enhancement • Behavior management: self-harm
• *Hopelessness*	• Decision making • Depression control • Hope • Mood equilibrium • Quality of life	• Decision-making support • Hope instillation • Mood management • Resiliency promotion • Self-modification assistance • Spiritual growth facilitation
• *Identity: personal, disturbed*	• Distorted thought control • Identity • Self-mutilation restraint	• Environmental management: violence protection • Self-esteem enhancement • Decision-making support
• *Self-esteem, chronic low*	• Depression level • Quality of life • Self-esteem	• Self-esteem enhancement • Mood management
• *Social isolation*	• Play participation • Social involvement • Social support • Well-being	• Behavior modification: social skills • Complex relationship building • Coping enhancement

(Continued)

- Recreation therapy
- Therapeutic play
- Socialization enhancement

• *Grieving,* *dysfunctional*	• Coping • Family coping • Grief resolution • Role performance	• Coping enhancement • Counseling • Family therapy • Grief work facilitation
• *Sorrow, chronic*	• Acceptance: health status • Depression control • Grief resolution	• Grief work facilitation • Spiritual support • Coping enhancement
• *Disturbed sleep* *pattern*	• Anxiety control • Comfort level • Psychosocial adjustment: life change • Rest • Sleep	• Coping enhancement • Energy management • Sleep enhancement

SCOLIOSIS

Brief Description

Scoliosis is a lateral curvature of the spine. Most cases are idiopathic in nature because there is no apparent cause, but there are also congenital and neuromuscular causes. Most common spinal deformity. Girls are more commonly affected. Usual age of onset is 10–11 years.

History and Physical Assessment
Findings

Child may complain of clothes not fitting well (e.g., uneven pant length). Otherwise, few obvious signs present at time of diagnosis. Child may exhibit asymmetry of shoulder height, scapula, or hip height. X ray studies and magnetic resonance imaging (MRI) are primary diagnostic tests used.

Nursing Care

Although controversial, screening programs are used with adolescents (by school nurses and at well-child visits). Early management consists of bracing (Boston brace, Milwaukee brace) and supplemental exercises. Noncompliance and body image disturbances are common with children who wear braces. Surgical correction (e.g., spinal fusion with Harrington rods, Luque instrumentation, or Cotrel-Dubousset procedure) required for severe curvatures.

Related Nursing Diagnoses	NOC Outcomes	NIC Interventions
• *Disturbed body image*	• Body image • Self-esteem	• Body image enhancement • Coping enhancement • Self-esteem enhancement
• *Mobility: physical, impaired*	• Body positioning • Ambulation • Joint movement	• Exercise promotion • Exercise therapy • Positioning
• *Skin integrity, risk for impaired*	• Tissue integrity: skin • Wound healing	• Skin surveillance • Wound care • Incision site care • Pressure management
• *Therapeutic regimen management, ineffective*	• Compliance behavior • Knowledge: treatment regimen	• Decision-making support • Patient contracting • Mutual goal setting • Teaching: procedure and treatment

SEIZURES

Brief Description

Seizures represent brief malfunctioning within the brain's electrical system. Abnormal electrical discharges from the brain cause paroxysmal, uncontrolled episodes of behavior. Common causes include CNS bleeding, CNS infection, metabolic abnormalities, head trauma, tumor, toxin ingestion, and fever. Seizures are usually idiopathic in nature.

Consequences of seizure activity can include alterations in responsiveness, in sensation and perception, and in movement and muscle tone. Seizures are classified as partial (i.e., limited to particular area of brain), generalized (i.e., involve both hemispheres of brain), or unclassified.

History and Physical Assessment Findings

Child and family should be asked to specifically describe seizure. Need to distinguish seizures from breath-holding spells. Careful seizure observation and documentation are necessary. Describe beginning of episode including any precipitating factors, including an aura. Also describe child's response to self and others. Clear description of movements, mobility, and tone is necessary. Include observation of exact location, indicating whether one or both sides of body are affected. Assessment is made for any postictal responses. Note how long it takes for child to resume previous activities. Results of CT scan, MRI, EEG, skull radiography, electromyogram (EMG), brain scan, lumbar puncture, and antiepileptic drug-blood levels should be noted.

Nursing Care

Prompt recognition of seizure activity is necessary to ensure safety. Stay with child during seizure. Protect child from potential injury (e.g., falls, aspiration pneumonia, hyperthermia). Be sure not to restrain child's movements. Reorient child after episode while providing reassurance and psychologic support for child and family. Emergency assistance should be sought if there is respiratory arrest or if seizure activity lasts for >5 min (status epilepticus), multiple seizure episodes occur without return of consciousness in between (status epilepticus), or child has sustained injury.

IV or PR administration of antiepileptic drugs such as diazepam, phenytoin, or phenobarbital are indicated during episodes of status epilepticus. Children usually are maintained on daily PO dosages of antiepileptic drugs. Client teaching regarding seizures, antiepileptic drugs, diagnostic testing, seizure recognition, and first aid is necessary.

Related Nursing Diagnoses	NOC Outcomes	NIC Interventions
• *Trauma, risk for*	• Knowledge: personal safety • Safety behavior: fall prevention • Safety behavior: personal	• Environmental management: safety • Fall prevention • Home maintenance assistance • Vital signs monitoring • Seizure precautions
• *Sensory perception, disturbed*	• Cognitive orientation • Sensory function • Neurological status	• Neurologic monitoring • Reality orientation • Environmental management • Surveillance: safety
• *Noncompliance (therapy), risk for*	• Adherence behavior • Compliance behavior • Symptom control • Treatment behavior: illness	• Health system guidance • Mutual goal setting • Patient contracting • Teaching: disease process

SEXUALLY TRANSMITTED DISEASES (STDs)

Chlamydial Infections

Infective Organism. Bacterium *Chlamydia trachomatis.*
Sources. Humans.
Transmission. Sexual.
Incubation Period. 8–21 days.

Signs and Symptoms. Urethritis, cervicitis, salpingitis, inguinal lymphadenopathy, vaginal discharge, dysuria, epididymitis, proctitis, lower abdominal pain, and menstrual irregularities. May be totally asymptomatic.

Diagnosis. Cell culture.

Nursing Care. PO antibiotics (e.g., doxycycline, azithromycin). Single-dose therapy preferred if possible. All sexual contacts should be treated. Follow-up therapy should be stressed. Reportable in most states.

Complications. Chronic conjunctivitis.

Gonorrhea

Infective Organism. *Neisseria gonorrhoeae*, gram-negative diplococcus.

Sources. Humans.

Transmission. Almost always sexually transmitted except in cases of vertical transmission from maternal cervix to conjunctiva of newborn.

Incubation Period. 2–6 days; in rare cases, 10–16 days.

Signs and Symptoms. Large percentage of clients asymptomatic. Clinical signs may include urethritis (males); cervicitis (females); pelvic inflammatory disease (PID); pharyngitis; and systemic complications of arthritis, dermatitis, meningitis, and endocarditis.

Diagnosis. Culture and Gram's stain. Patients with gonorrhea should be screened for other STDs.

Nursing Care. Single injection or oral dose of antibiotics (e.g., ceftriaxone or cefixime). All sexual contacts should be treated. Important to stress treatment to prevent long-term complications. Prevention strategies encouraged (e.g., case finding, public health education, use of condoms and spermacide). Mandatory reporting required.

Complications. Genitourinary problems in males, occlusion of fallopian tubes in females, sterility.

Herpes Simplex Virus Type 2 (HSV-2)

Infective Organism. Herpes simplex virus type 2 (HSV-2).

Sources. Humans.

Transmission. Through contact with lesions.

Incubation Period. 2–12 days.

Signs and Symptoms. Presentation ranges from asymptomatic to systemic illness. Single lesion or cluster of papules can appear on genitalia, thighs, or buttocks. Papules develop into vesicles and pustules and eventually become ulcerations. Intense pain and itching occur when ulcers break. Area lymph nodes enlarge frequently.

Diagnosis. Viral culture.

Nursing Care. Acyclovir (PO) is drug of choice. Oral sex should be discouraged if lesions are in mouth or on lips, vagina, or penis. Anal intercourse should be discouraged when lesions are active. Lesions should be washed with soap and water to prevent secondary infection. Condom use recommended. Immunocompromised clients at risk for systemic infection. Sexual partners with lesions should be treated. Increased risk for HIV in those with open lesions.

Complications. Encephalitis, herpes simplex keratitis, gingivostomatitis.

Human Papilloma Virus (HPV)

Infective Organism. Human papilloma virus (HPV).

Sources. Humans.

Transmission. Sexual contact; precursor to cancer of cervix. Perinatal transmission to infants.

Incubation Period. 1–6 months.

Signs and Symptoms. Condyloma acuminatum (wart with cauliflower-like appearance) located on genitalia, around anus, or in mouth. Size varies from several millimeters to several centimeters.

Diagnosis. Physical examination and viral cultures.

Nursing Care. No cure exists. Virus controlled by podofilox or interferon. Warts can be removed by cryotherapy or laser surgery.

Syphilis

Infective Organism. *Spirochaeta pallida/Treponema pallidum.*

Sources. Humans.

Transmission. Congenital transmission to fetus; otherwise, transmitted sexually.

Incubation Period. 10–90 days; most infectious during first year of disease.

Signs and Symptoms. Chancre in anogenital region, rash, general malaise, condyloma latum papules on moist areas of skin. Congenital—mucocutaneous lesions, snuffles, hepatosplenomegaly, lymphadenopathy, and failure to thrive. Infant also may be asymptomatic.

Diagnosis. Serologic tests for Venereal Disease Research Laboratory (VDRL) and rapid plasma reagent (RPR).

Nursing Care. Congenital syphilis—penicillin G for 10–14 days. Acquired syphilis—penicillin G IM, doxycycline PO, or tetracycline PO depending on age of child and duration of disease. All sexual partners should be contacted, evaluated, and treated. Clients should have repeat VDRL 3, 6, and 12 months after therapy. Mandatory reporting required.

SICKLE CELL ANEMIA

Brief Description

Sickle cell anemia is a hereditary hemoglobinopathy in which there is partial or complete replacement of normal hemoglobin with abnormal hemoglobin S. This is an autosomal-recessive disorder. Therefore, if both parents have the sickle cell trait, there is a 25% chance that offspring will have the disease. It occurs most in those of African descent and occasionally affects people of Mediterranean descent.

Hemoglobin in RBCs acquires an elongated crescent or sickle shape. These cells are more rigid and obstruct capillary blood flow, leading to tissue ischemia. Organs become scarred from damaged tissue. Sickling is triggered by events such as fever, stress, dehydration, and hypoxia. Sickled cells resume a more normal shape with hydration and oxygenation; however, cell membrane is more fragile and cell life is only 10–20 days versus normal 120 days.

History and Physical Assessment Findings

Symptoms generally do not appear until 4–6 months of age because of the presence of fetal hemoglobin. Diagnosis is made by hemoglobin electrophoresis through newborn screening. Results in shortened life span of blood vessels. Also tissue destruction, which results from vaso-occlusion.

Changes occur in most body systems, although the most common signs and symptoms include the following:

- Brain—headache; convulsion; visual problems (indicative of cerebrovascular accident)
- Eyes—diminished vision as a result of retinopathy; retinal detachment
- Skin—decreased peripheral circulation leading to leg ulcers
- Extremities—peripheral neuropathy; weakness; arthralgia
- Bones—susceptibility to infection as a result of chronic ischemia
- Liver—engorgement and scarring
- Spleen—fibrosis of spleen leading to increased number of infections

There are three types of sickle cell crisis:

1. Vaso-occlusive—most common type; painful; caused by stasis of blood with cell clumping in microcirculation, ischemia, infarction; fever, pain, and tissue engorgement are common signs
2. Splenic sequestration—life-threatening crisis; caused by pooling of blood within spleen; anemia, hypovolemia, and shock are common signs
3. Aplastic crisis—reduced production and increased destruction of RBCs; crisis usually triggered by viral infection; anemia and pallor are common signs

Nursing Care

No cure for sickle cell anemia. Nursing care should aim at prevention and treatment of sickling episodes. Prevention strategies include avoiding exposure to infections, maintaining adequate hydration, promptly treating infections, and maintaining routine health visits. For children experiencing sickle cell crises, treatment includes hydration restoration, supplemental oxygenation, pain management, treatment or prevention of infection, and bed rest. Children may require blood transfusions to treat anemia.

Related Nursing Diagnoses	NOC Outcomes	NIC Interventions
• *Acute pain*	• Comfort level • Pain: disruptive effects	• Medication management • Analgesic administration • Patient-controlled analgesia assistance • Pain management • Presence • Relaxation therapy • Distraction • Heat application • Music therapy • Guided imagery
• *Knowledge, deficient*	• Knowledge: prevention and prescribed medication • Knowledge: treatment regimen	• Teaching: disease process • Teaching: prescribed medication • Risk identification • Parent education: childrearing family
• *Tissue perfusion, ineffective (cardiopulmonary and cerebral)*	• Tissue perfusion: pulmonary • Tissue perfusion: cerebral	• Oxygen therapy • Respiratory monitoring • Positioning • Blood products administration

SLIPPED CAPITAL FEMORAL EPIPHYSIS (SCFE)

Brief Description

SCFE, a displacement (abrupt or gradual) of the proximal femoral epiphysis, usually develops during accelerated periods of growth (preadolescent and adolescent) and is more common in obese children. Although cause is unknown, SCFE is thought to be influenced by hormonal factors (growth hormone, sex hormones). Also associated with endocrine disorders such as hypothyroidism and growth hormone deficiency.

History and Physical Assessment Findings

Child usually reports limp and acute pain in groin, thigh, or knee. Hip range of motion (ROM) is painful and limited. X ray studies demonstrate altered position of femoral head.

Nursing Care

Assessment of child's ROM, pain, and limp is necessary. Before treatment, it is essential that child keep weight off affected joint. Children with SCFE require surgical intervention (fixation with screws or pins). Nursing management requires caring for child in traction, administering analgesics and other pain-reduction interventions, educating child and family about disorder, and promoting compliance with medical regimen.

Related Nursing Diagnoses	NOC Outcomes	NIC Interventions
• *Acute pain*	• Comfort level • Pain control • Pain: disruptive effects	• Analgesic administration • Pain management • Patient-controlled analgesia (PCA) assitance
• *Mobility: physical, impaired*	• Ambulation • Joint movement • Body positioning • Transfer performance	• Exercise therapy • Positioning
• *Risk for infection*	• Infection status • Knowledge: infection control • Wound healing	• Infection control • Infection protection • Incision site care • Wound care

SUBSTANCE ABUSE

Brief Description

Most adolescents have some experience with an illicit drug by the time they are high school seniors. Some of these adolescents progress to dependence. Risk factors include any of the following factors: family history of alcoholism or use of other drugs, history of family conflict, history of physical or sexual abuse, antisocial behavior, academic underachievement, low self-esteem, peers who use drugs, and early first use of illicit drugs. Often, substance abuse progresses from use of beer, wine, and tobacco to liquor to marijuana to cocaine or heroin. Many adolescents use multiple drugs simultaneously.

Some commonly abused substances include alcohol, marijuana and other cannabis substances, CNS depressants such as barbiturates, CNS stimulants such as amphetamines, cocaine, hallucinogens such as lysergic acid diethylamide (LSD), opioids such as morphine and heroin, and volatile substances such as hydrocarbons and nitrous oxide.

History and Physical Assessment Findings

Be alert to history findings consistent with personality changes, unexplained behavior or behavior out of the ordinary, poor family interaction, deteriorating school performance, and withdrawal from regular activities (e.g., sports, extracurricular activities, church). Injuries related to falls, fights, and motor vehicle accidents also should alert you to the possibility of substance abuse. The majority of youth who attempt suicide have history of many years of substance abuse.

Nursing Care

Treatment of drug toxicity or withdrawal depends on actual drug used. Long-term rehabilitation often requires adolescent to be withdrawn from both the environment and the actual chemical. May involve treatment programs such as Alcoholics Anonymous, Narcotics Anonymous, and other similar 12-step programs. Nurses must also play a major role in prevention programs.

Related Nursing Diagnoses	NOC Outcomes	NIC Interventions
• *Family processes, interrupted*	• Family coping • Family functioning	• Coping enhancement • Family support • Counseling • Family therapy • Support group • Role enhancement • Behavior modification
• *Denial, ineffective*	• Acceptance: health status • Symptom control	• Counseling • Decision-making support • Self-awareness enhancement • Self-responsibility facilitation • Behavior modification
• *Injury, risk for*	• Safety status: physical injury	• Surveillance: safety • Environmental management: safety • Risk identification

(Continued)

Related Nursing Diagnoses	NOC Outcomes	NIC Interventions
• *Sensory perceptions, disturbed: visual, auditory, or tactile*	• Cognitive orientation	• Hallucination management • Anxiety reduction • Medication management • Environmental management • Reality orientation • Substance use treatment
• *Nutrition, imbalanced: less than body requirements*	• Nutritional status: food and fluid intake • Nutritional status: nutrient intake	• Nutrition monitoring • Nutritional counseling • Medication management • Laboratory data interpretation
• *Knowledge, deficient*	• Knowledge: medication	• Teaching: prescribed medication
• *Violence: other-directed, risk for*	• Abusive behavior self-control • Aggression control • Distorted thought control • Impulse control • Risk control: alcohol use • Risk control: drug use	• Environmental management: violence prevention • Impulse control training
• *Violence: self-directed, risk for*	• Depression control • Distorted thought control • Impulse control • Suicide self-restraint	• Behavior management: self-harm • Environmental management: violence prevention • Suicide prevention

ULCERATIVE COLITIS (UC)
Brief Description

UC is considered a chronic inflammatory bowel disease characterized by exacerbations and remissions. Etiology is multifactorial in nature and thought to involve infectious organisms, dietary habits, genetic susceptibility, and environmental toxins. Most severely affected sites are the colon and rectum. Areas become ulcerated and edematous. Continous segments of bowel are affected at both mucosa and submucosa layers.

History and Physical Assessment Findings

Symptoms often include bloody diarrhea, intense abdominal pain, and weight loss. Diarrhea is often severe. Medical diagnosis is based on history, physical findings, laboratory tests (e.g., CBC, sedimentation rate, total protein, albumin, stool occult blood), and other diagnostic tests (e.g., upper GI, barium enema, endoscopy, sigmoidoscopy, colonoscopy, rectal biopsy, CT scan).

Nursing Care

Pharmacologic treatment for UC involves drugs that control inflammation. Corticosteroids are the most effective medication. Nutritional support is the paramount concern in children with UC because of growth retardation. Both enteral and parenteral nutritional support may be necessary. Children with UC need a well-balanced, high-protein, and high-calorie diet. Frequently a need exists for supplemental multivitamins, iron, and folic acid. Surgery may be indicated in clients who do not respond well to medical and nutritional approaches.

Related Nursing Diagnoses	NOC Outcomes	NIC Interventions
• *Fluid volume, deficient*	• Fluid balance	• Fluid management • Electrolyte monitoring • Laboratory data interpretation • Total parenteral nutrition • Hemorrhage control
• *Risk for infection*	• Infection status • Safety status: physical injury	• Infection protection • Laboratory data interpretation • Medication administration • Specimen management • Vital signs monitoring
• *Acute pain*	• Comfort level • Pain control	• Pain management • Coping enhancement • Distraction
• *Nausea*	• Comfort level • Hydration • Symptom severity	• Fluid/electrolyte management • Nausea management • Medication management • Vomiting management

(*Continued*)

Related Nursing Diagnoses	NOC Outcomes	NIC Interventions
• *Diarrhea*	• Electrolyte and acid-base balance • Symptom severity	• Fluid/electrolyte management • Diarrhea management • Laboratory data interpretation • Anxiety reduction • Medication administration
• *Skin integrity, impaired, risk for (perineal/perianal area)*	• Tissue integrity: skin and mucous membranes	• Bathing • Bowel incontinence care • Skin care: topical treatments • Diarrhea management • Perineal care • Self-care assistance • Bathing/hygiene
• *Knowledge, deficient*	• Knowledge: medication • Knowledge: disease process	• Teaching: prescribed medication • Teaching: disease process

URINARY TRACT INFECTION (UTI)
Brief Description

Urinary tract infection is primarily caused by *Escherichia coli* and other gram-negative enteric pathogens. Other causative pathogens include *Proteus* species, enterococci, *Klebsiella* species, *S. aureus*, and *Pseudomonas* species. Anatomic, physical, and chemical conditions and urinary tract properties are factors that contribute to development of UTI. Urinary stasis is the most common host factor. UTIs are more commonly seen in females because of their short urethra and its proximity to the anus.

History and Physical Assessment Findings

Common assessment findings include dysuria, frequency, urgency, costovertebral angle tenderness, and enuresis. Nonspecific findings such as vomiting, diarrhea, fever, and lethargy also may be present. It should be noted that some UTIs are asymptomatic, especially in infants and very young children. Positive urine culture confirms diagnosis. Diagnostic tests such as voiding cystourethrogram (VCUG) may be necessary to detect anatomic defects. Other commonly performed diagnostic tests include ultrasonography and intravenous pyelogram (IVP).

Nursing Care

Depending on culture and sensitivity results, specific antibiotics are administered. Penicillins, sulfonamides, cephalosporins, and tetracyclines are the most commonly prescribed antibiotics for UTIs. Route of administration usually is PO unless child has pyelonephritis, in which case IV route is used. Antipyretics are used to decrease fever. Renal ultrasound and VCUG may be ordered to rule out any anatomic problems after infection is cleared. Child and family may need education regarding prevention (e.g., practicing proper hygiene, avoiding bubble baths, wearing cotton underwear) and treatment of infection.

Related Nursing Diagnoses	NOC Outcomes	NIC Interventions
• *Urinary elimination, impaired*	• Urinary elimination	• Urinary elimination management
• *Hyperthermia*	• Thermoregulation	• Fever treatment • Vital signs monitoring
• *Acute pain*	• Comfort level • Pain control	• Analgesic administration • Pain management
• *Injury, risk for*	• Risk control • Safety behavior: personal	• Environmental management: safety • Health education
• *Knowledge, deficient*	• Knowledge: disease process	• Teaching: disease process • Teaching: prescribed medication

URTICARIA
Brief Description

Urticaria generally represents an allergic response to drugs or infection. May be accompanied by general malaise, fever, and lymphadenopathy. Severe reactions may involve internal organs and joints. Obstruction of the airway constitutes a medical emergency. Multiple etiologies, but often cause is not identified. Some common causes are drugs (e.g., penicillin, acetylsalicylic acid), food (e.g., peanuts, milk, shellfish, food additives), insect bites, infection, heat, and animal dander. Urticaria may occur as acute, chronic, or recurrent attack.

History and Physical Assessment Findings

Cause for urticaria is often unknown. Family members and child should be questioned regarding exposure to any of the previously noted common causes. Lesions usually are circular wheals with well-circumscribed borders, but can be of variable size and shape. They tend to appear quickly. Lesions may be localized or generalized and may include swelling of the tongue. Any obstruction of air passages requires emergent medical treatment.

Nursing Care

Antihistamines (e.g., hydroxyzine hydrochloride [Atarax], diphenhydramine hydrochloride [Benadryl]) prescribed for urticaria. If severe, oral prednisone may be prescribed. If clients experience recurrent acute episodes, an EpiPen kit (for auto-injection of epinephrine) should be carried. If possible, families should try to identify and avoid allergens.

Related Nursing Diagnoses	NOC Outcomes	NIC Interventions
• *Injury, risk for*	• Immune status • Risk control	• Allergy management • Environmental management: safety • Latex precautions • Risk identification
• *Pain*	• Comfort level • Pain control	• Medication management
• *Knowledge, deficient*	• Knowledge: allergen prevention • Knowledge: treatment regimen	• Teaching: disease process • Teaching: prescribed medication

CHAPTER 7

CLINICAL REFERENCES AND RESOURCES

PEDIATRIC NURSING JOURNALS

Issues in Comprehensive Pediatric Nursing

Published by Taylor & Francis Group
325 Chestnut Street, Suite 800
Philadelphia, PA 19106
1-215-625-8900

Journal of Pediatric Health Care (Official Journal of the National Association of Pediatric Nurse Associates and Practitioners)

Published by Elsevier
11830 Westline Industrial Drive
St. Louis, MO 63146
1-314-453-4100

Journal of Pediatric Nursing (Official Journal of the Society of Pediatric Nurses)

Published by Elsevier
11830 Westline Industrial Drive
St. Louis, MO 63146
1-314-453-4100

Journal of Pediatric Oncology Nursing

Published by Sage Publications
2455 Teller Road
Thousand Oaks, CA 91320
1-800-818-7243

Journal for Specialists in Pediatric Nursing

Published by Blackwell Publishing
350 Main Street
Malden, MA 02148
1-781-388-8200

MCN: The American Journal of Maternal/Child Nursing

Published by Lippincott Williams & Wilkins
351 W Camden Street
Baltimore, MD 21201
1-410-528-4000

Pediatric Nursing

Published by Jannetti Publications, Inc.
East Holly Avenue
Box 56
Pitman, NJ 08071-0056
1-856-256-2300

RESOURCES FOR CHILD-HEALTH NURSING

General Child Health Resources

American Academy of Pediatrics
141 Northwest Point Boulevard
Elk Grove Village, IL 60007-1098
1-847-434-4000
http://www.aap.org

Centers for Disease Control and Prevention (CDC)
1600 Clifton Road
Atlanta, GA 30333
1-800-311-3435
http://www.cdc.gov

Information for children and families
http://www.kidshealth.org

National Immunization Hotline (at the CDC)
National Immunization Program (NIP)
1600 Clifton Road, NE
Atlanta, GA 30333
1-800-CDC-INFO
1-800-232-4636
http://www.cdc.gov

National Parent to Parent Support and Information System, Inc. (NPPSIS)
P.O. Box 907
Blue Ridge, GA 30513
1-706-632-8822
http://www.iser.com

National Safe Kids
1301 Pennsylvania Avenue, NW
Suite 1000
Washington, DC 20004
1-202-662-0600
http://www.safekids.org

AIDS/HIV Resources

AIDS Information Hotline
CDC-INFO
1-800-CDC-INFO
http://www.cdc.gov

Elizabeth Glaser Pediatric AIDS Foundation
1140 Connecticut Avenue, NW
Suite 200
Washington, DC 20036
1-202-296-9165
http://www.pedaids.org

National Pediatric AIDS Network
P.O. Box 1032
Boulder, CO 80306
http://www.npan.org

National Pediatric and Family HIV Resource Center
1-800-362-0071
http://www.pedhivaids.org

Women, Children, and HIV Resources for Prevention and Treatment
http://www.womenchildrenhiv.org

Asthma/Allergy Resources

Allergy and Asthma Network Mothers of Asthmatics
2751 Prosperity Avenue
Suite 150
Fairfax, VA 22031
1-800-878-4403
http://www.aanma.org

American Academy of Allergy, Asthma, and Immunology
555 East Wells Street
Suite 1100
Milwaukee, WI 53202-3823
1-414-272-6071
http://www.aaaai.org

American College of Allergy, Asthma, and Immunology
85 West Algonquin Road
Suite 550
Arlington Heights, IL 60005
http://www.acaai.org

American Lung Association
61 Broadway, 6th Floor
New York, NY 10006
1-800-LUNGUSA
1-800-548-8252
http://www.lungusa.org

Asthma and Allergy Foundation of America
1233 20th Street, NW, Suite 402
Washington, D.C. 20036
1-202-466-7643
http://www.aafa.org

CDC National Center for Environmental Health
http://www.cdc.gov

National Heart, Lung, and Blood Institute
NHLBI Health Information Center
P.O. Box 30105
Bethesda, MD 20824-0105
1-301-592-8576
http://www.nhlbi.nih.gov

National Library of Medicine and the National Institutes of Health
8600 Rockville Pike
Bethesda, MD 20894
http://www.nlm.nih.gov

Birth Defects/Special Needs Children Resources

Birth Defect Research for Children
930 Woodcock Road, Suite 225
Orlando, FL 32803
1-407-895-0802
http://www.birthdefects.org

Blind Children's Center
4120 Marathon Street
Los Angeles, CA 90029
1-323-664-2153
http://www.blindcntr.org

Deafness Research Foundation
8201 Greensboro Drive
Suite 300
McLean, VA 22102
1-800-829-5934
http://drf.org

March of Dimes Birth Defects Foundation
1275 Mamaroneck Avenue
White Plains, NY 10605
1-888-663-4637
http://www.modimes.org

National Down Syndrome Society
666 Broadway
New York, NY 10012
1-800-221-4602
http://www.ndss.org

National Easter Seals Society for Crippled Children
230 West Monroe Street, Suite 1800
Chicago, IL 60606
1-312-726-6200
http://www.easter-seals.org

United Cerebral Palsy Association
UCP National
1660 L Street NW, Suite 700
Washington, DC 20036-5602
1-800-USA-5UCP
http://www.ucpa.org

Cancer Resources

American Cancer Society
1-800-ACS-2345
http://www.cancer.org

The Leukemia & Lymphoma Society
600 Third Avenue
New York, NY 10016
1-800-955-4572
http://www.leukemia.org

National Cancer Institute
NIH Building 31, Room 10A03
31 Center Drive MSC 2580
Bethesda, MD 20892-2580
1-800-4-CANCER
http://www.nci.nih.gov

Diabetes/Renal Resources

American Diabetes Association
1701 North Beauregard Street
Alexandria, VA 22311
1-800-DIABETES
http://www.diabetes.org

Juvenile Diabetes Foundation International
120 Wall Street
New York, NY 10005-4001
1-800-533-CURE (2873)
http://www.jdf.org

National Kidney Foundation
30 East 33rd Street, Suite 1100
New York, NY 10016
1-800-622-9010
http://www.kidney.org

Drug Abuse Resources

National Council on Alcoholism and Drug Dependence
20 Exchange Place
Suite 2902
New York, NY 10005
1-800-475-HOPE

National Institute of Drug Abuse
6001 Executive Boulevard
Room 5213
Bethesda, MD 20892
1-301-443-1124
http://www.nida.nih.gov

U.S. Department of Health and Human Services
Center for Substance Abuse Treatment
1-800-662-HELP
http://www.samhsa.gov

U.S. Department of Health and Human Services and National Clearing
 House for Alcohol and Drug Information
1-800-729-6686
http://www.health.org

Heart Disease Resources

American Heart Association
National Center
7272 Greenville Avenue
Dallas, TX 75231-4596
1-800-242-8721
http://www.americanheart.org

Congenital Heart Information Network
1561 Clark Drive
Yardley, PA 19067
1-215-493-3068
http://www.tchin.org

Mental Health Resources

American Anorexia/Bulimia Association
165 West 46th Street, Suite 1108
New York, NY 10036
1-800-522-2230

Autism Society of America
7910 Woodmont Avenue
Suite 300
Bethesda, MD 20814-3067
1-301-657-0881
http://www.autism-society.org

Children and Adults with Attention-Deficit/Hyperactivity Disorder
8181 Professional Place
Suite 150
Landover, MD 20785
1-800-233-4050
http://www.chadd.org

National Association of Anorexia Nervosa and Associated Disorders
P.O. Box 7
Highland Park, IL 60035
1-847-831-3438
http://www.anad.org

National Attention Deficit Disorder Association
P.O. Box 543
Pottstown, PA 19464
1-484-945-2101
http://www.add.org

National Mental Health Association
2001 N. Beauregard Street, 12th Floor
Alexandria, VA 22311
1-800-969-6642
http://www.nmha.org

Other Resources

American Burn Association
625 N. Michigan Avenue, Suite 2550
Chicago, IL 60611
1-312-642-9260
http://www.ameriburn.org

American Cleft Palate-Craniofacial Association (CPF)
1504 East Franklin Street
Suite 102
Chapel Hill, NC 27514-2820
1-919-933-9044
http://www.cleftline.org

Brain Injury Association of America
8201 Greensboro Drive
Suite 611
McLean, VA 22102
1-703-761-0750
http://www.biausa.org

Crohn's and Colitis Foundation of America
386 Park Avenue South
17th Floor
New York, NY 10016
1-800-932-2423
http://www.ccfa.org

Cystic Fibrosis Foundation
6931 Arlington Road
Bethesda, MD 20814
1-800-FIGHTCF
http://www.cff.org

Epilepsy Foundation
4351 Garden City Drive
Landover, MD 20785
1-800-EFA-1000
http://www.efa.org

First Candle/Sudden Infant Death Syndrome (SIDS) Alliance
1-800-221-7437
1314 Bedford Avenue, Suite 210
Baltimore, MD 21208
1-410-653-8226
http://www.sidsalliance.org

National Attention Deficit Disorder Association
1788 Second Street, Suite 200
Highland Park, IL 60035
1-847-432-ADDA

National Clearinghouse on Child Abuse and Neglect Information
330 C Street, SW
Washington, DC 20447
1-800-394-3366
http://nccanch.acf.hhs.gov

National Hemophilia Foundation
116 W. 32nd Street, 11th Fl.
New York, NY 10001
1-800-42-HANDI
http://www.hemophilia.org

National Organization of Rare Disorders, Inc.
55 Kenosia Ave.
P.O. Box 1968
Danbury, CT
06813-1968
(203) 744-0100
http://www.rarediseases.org

National Pediculosis Association
50 Kearney Road
Needham, MA 02494
1-781-449-NITS
http://www.headlice.org

Neurofibromatosis Foundation
95 Pine Street, 16th Floor
New York, NY 10005
1-800-323-7938
http://www.nf.org

Sickle Cell Disease Association of America
16 S. Calvert Street
Suite 600
Baltimore, MD 21202
1-800-421-8453
http://www.sicklecelldisease.org

EVALUATING THE CREDIBILITY OF HEALTH INFORMATION FOUND ON THE INTERNET

Nurses, as well as patients and families, are utilizing the Internet with increasing frequency to learn more about health and illness. Although the Internet provides an explosion of health information at one's fingertips, it is important that nurses understand how to evaluate the credibility of health information found on the Internet. Nurses must also teach patients this very important skill.

Nicoll (2000, 2001) describes a simple mnemonic, "Are you PLEASED with the site?" to illustrate seven website evaluation criteria. In order to determine if you are PLEASED, it is important to consider the following areas.

P (Purpose)	• What is the author's purpose in developing the site? • Is there congruence between the author's purpose and your purpose for using this site?
L (Links)	• Do the links in this site connect to reliable sites? Do they all work?
E (Editorial)	• Is the information in the site accurate, comprehensive, and current? • Is there any bias in the information provided? • Are there misspellings or grammatical errors?
A (Author)	• Who is the author of the site? What are his or her credentials? • Does the site identify by name the author and contact information? • Is the author associated with a reputable organization or institution? (Remember that anyone can post a website and can present himself or herself in any way)
S (Site)	• Is the site easy to navigate? • Is it attractive?
E (Ethical)	• Is there contact information for the site developer and author? • Is there full disclosure as to the purpose of the site?
D (Date)	• When was the site last updated? • Is it current?

Nicoll, L. (2000). Quick and effectice website evaluation. *Computers in Nursing*, 3(3), 9.
Nicoll, L. (2001). *Nurses' guide to the Internet* (3rd ed.). Philadelphia: J.B. Lippincott.

REFERENCES

American Academy of Pediatrics. (1994). *Toy safety: Guidelines for parents*. Elk Grove Village, IL: American Academy of Pediatrics.

Behrman, R., Kliegman, R., Jenson, H., & Kliegman, R. (2003). *Nelson textbook of pediatrics* (17th ed.). Philadelphia: Elsevier Mosby.

Betz, C., & Sowden, L. (2004). *Mosby's pediatric nursing reference*. Philadelphia: Elsevier Mosby.

Centers for Disease Control and Prevention. (1994). Revised classification system for human immunodeficiency virus infection in children less than 13 years of age. *Morbidity and Morality Weekly Report, 43*, 1–10 (MMWR No. RR-12).

Centers for Disease Control and Prevention. (1997). *Preventing lead poisoning in young children*. Atlanta: Author.

Corbett, J.V. (2003). *Laboratory tests and diagnostic procedures with nursing diagnoses* (6th ed.). Upper Saddle River, NJ: Prentice Hall.

Estes, M. (2002). *Health assessment & physical examination* (2nd ed.). Clifton Park, NY: Thomson Delmar Learning.

Estes, M. (2006). *Health assessment & physical examination* (3rd ed.). Clifton Park, NY: Thomson Delmar Learning

Frankenburg, W.K. & Dodds, J.B. (1990). *Denver II*. Denver: Denver Developmental Materials, Inc.

Giger, J. & Davidhizar, R. (1999). *Transcultural nursing: Assessment and intervention* (3rd ed.). Baltimore: Mosby.

Giger, J., & Davidhizar, R. (2004). *Transcultural nursing: Assessment and intervention* (4th ed.). Baltimore: Mosby.

Gunn, V., Nechyba, C., & Johns Hopkins Hospital Children's Medical and Surgical Center. (2003). *The Harriet Lane Handbook: A manual for pediatric house officers*. Philadelphia: Elsevier Mosby.

Hockenberry, M. (2005). *Wong's essentials of pediatric nursing* (7th ed.). Philadelphia: Elsevier Mosby.

Kemper, K.J. (1997). A practical approach to chronic asthma management. *Contemporary Pediatrics, 14*(8), 86–114.

La Leche League. (2005). Human milk storage information. Available at http://www.lalecheleague.org/FAQ/milkstorage.html

Mandleco, B. (2005). *Pediatric nursing skills & procedures*. Clifton Park, NY: Thomson Delmar Learning.

Merkel, S., Voepel-Lewis, T., Shayevitz, J., & Malviya, S. (1997). The FLACC: A behavioral scale for scoring postoperative pain in young children. *Pediatric Nursing, 23*(3), 293–297.

National Association of State Public Interest Research Groups. (2004). Trouble in toyland: The 19th annual survey of toy safety. Retrieved from http://www.toysafety.net.

National Institutes of Health. (1997). *Guidelines for the diagnosis and management of asthma: National asthma education program—expert panel report*. Bethesda, MD: Author.

Nicoll, L. (2000). Quick and effective website evaluation. *Computers in Nursing, 3*(3), 9.

Nicoll, L. (2001). *Nurses' guide to the Internet* (3rd ed.). Philadelphia: J.B. Lippincott.

Pickering, L. (2003). *2003 Red Book: Report of the Committee on Infectious Diseases*. Elk Grove Village, IL: American Academy of Pediatrics.

Potts, N.L. & Mandleco, B. (2002). *Pediatric nursing: Caring for children and their families*. Clifton Park, NY: Thomson Delmar Learning.

Potts, N. L., & Mandleco, B. (2007). *Pediatric nursing: Caring for children and their families* (2nd ed.). Clifton Park, NY: Thomson Delmar Learning.

Ramsey, S. (2000). Abusive situations. In S. Killion & K. Dempski, *Quick look nursing: Legal and ethical issues*. Thorofare, NJ: Slack Incorporated.

Rush, S., & Harr, J. (2001). Evidence-based pediatric nursing: Does it have to hurt? *AACN Clinical Issues, 12*(4), 597–605.

Schwartz, M. W. (2003). *Clinical handbook of pediatrics* (3rd ed.). Philadelphia: Lippincott, Williams & Wilkins.

Swearingen, P. (2004). *All-in-one care planning resource*. Philadelphia: Elsevier Mosby.

Taketomo, C. K., Hodding, J. H., & Kraus, D. M. (2004). *Pediatric dosage handbook* (11th ed.). Hudson, OH: Lexi-Comp, Incorporated.

U.S. Department of Agriculture, Center for Nutrition Policy and Promotion. (2005). *MyPyramid: Steps to a healthier you*. Retrieved from http://www.mypyramid.gov.

Wilkinson, J. (2005). *Prentice Hall nursing diagnosis handbook* (8th ed.). Upper Saddle River, NJ: Prentice Hall.

INDEX